ACSM
Health & Fitness Track
Certification Study Guide 2000

ACSM Exercise Leader®

ACSM Health/Fitness InstructorSM

ACSM Health/Fitness Director®

**Prepared by the ACSM
Health/Fitness Subcommittee
of the Committee on Certification
and Education**

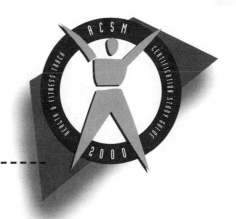

American College of Sports Medicine

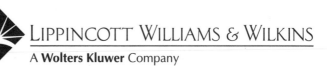
LIPPINCOTT WILLIAMS & WILKINS
A **Wolters Kluwer** Company

To purchase additional copies of this book, call our customer service department at **(800) 638-3030** or fax orders to **(301) 824-7390.** International customers should call **(301) 714-2324.** Or visit **Lippincott Williams & Wilkins on the Internet: http://www.lww.com.**

For more information concerning American College of Sports Medicine certification and suggested preparatory materials, call **(800) 486-5643** or visit the American College of Sports Medicine Website at **www.acsm.org.**

00 01 02 03 04
2 3 4 5 6 7 8 9 10

Contents

Valid 2000 and 2001

ACSM HEALTH/FITNESS DIRECTOR® CERTIFICATION   61

APPENDIX A   71

General Information

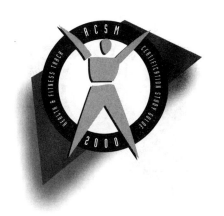

This study guide is designed to help qualified individuals prepare for the American College of Sports Medicine (ACSM) Health & Fitness Track certifications. The Health & Fitness Track is designed primarily for leaders of preventive health programs in corporate, commercial, and community settings aimed at apparently healthy individuals or persons with controlled diseases. There are three levels of certification that comprise the Health & Fitness Track: ACSM Exercise Leader®, ACSM Health/Fitness Instructor_SM, and ACSM Health/Fitness Director®.

The certification process is designed to evaluate competence in the ACSM knowledge, skills, and abilities (KSAs) found in Appendix F of the 6th edition of *ACSM's Guidelines for Exercise Testing and Prescription.*

HOW TO USE THIS GUIDE

The certification study guide is intended as a resource for some of the information that will be potentially used in the certification exam. This guide will help the candidate understand the format for the written and practical exams and provide much of the relevant information, including protocols that will be used in the workshops and exams. This study guide is not intended to completely prepare the candidate for the health/fitness certifications, but to provide information and resources to help in the overall preparation for the certifications. It is recommended that candidates supplement the use of this study guide with other preparatory materials. A bibliography at the end of each certification provides additional recommended resources for studying.

It is recommended that the candidate initially determine which certification level is appropriate for his/her skills and goals. To determine the appropriate level, the candidate should first review the minimum requirements and recommended competencies and decide which level or levels one may qualify for. The next step is to complete the sample tests to assess the level of knowledge for the certification level. If the candidate scores less than 50% correct, consideration should be given to a lower level certification.

It is important to note that the ACSM Health/Fitness Instructor_SM candidate is responsible for all of the information and KSAs of both the ACSM Exercise Leader® and the ACSM Health/Fitness Instructor_SM levels, and the ACSM Health/Fitness Director® is responsible for the information and KSAs of all three levels in the Health/Fitness Track.

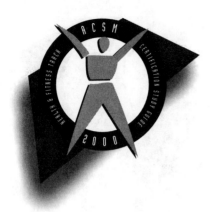

WORKSHOP INFORMATION

ACSM workshops may be conducted before certifications. Workshops are optional and are not a prerequisite for certification. ACSM workshops are designed to develop and enhance the knowledge base and practical skills of the participants. The curriculum has been developed so that didactic material and its practical application are scheduled in concert. In this way, the participant is better able to assimilate theory and practice.

In addition to the recommended prerequisites, participants should have adequate knowledge and background in the health and fitness profession. The workshops are not intended to provide the full experience and knowledge necessary for ACSM certification.

CERTIFICATION INFORMATION

The ACSM certifications encompass cognitive and practical competencies that are evaluated in both written and practical examination components. The candidate must successfully complete both written and practical components to receive ACSM certification. Additionally, current cardiopulmonary resuscitation (CPR) certification is required to maintain ACSM certification. This study guide contains information for the three levels of certification that comprise the Health & Fitness Track.

Written Examination

The written examination for each level of certification is composed of approximately 115 multiple choice questions drawn from the KSAs found in the 6th edition of *ACSM's Guidelines for Exercise Testing and Prescription*. Candidates are given 3 hours to complete the written examination and must present a valid picture identification to be admitted to take the examination. Candidates should refer to the certification level they are interested in for a more detailed discussion of the written examination. Candidates are advised that each examination will contain approximately 15 randomly distributed questions that are being "tested" for use in future examinations. These questions will be scored; however, they will not be counted in the final results. The candidate's score will be based on approximately 100 multiple choice questions.

This study guide contains sample examination questions similar to those found on the written examination. These sample questions are intended to illustrate the depth of knowledge expected for each level of certification. The time limitation is strictly enforced. The written examination is scored through the ACSM National Center. Certification sites do not have test results.

Practical Examination

Each certification level contains a practical examination component that uses examination stations. Competencies for the practical examination are also based on the KSAs. Each station has an objective checklist of skills, actions, and responses to testing situations on which the examiner documents the results. Time limitations are strictly enforced. The practical examination is then scored at the ACSM National Center. Certification sites do not have test results.

During the practical examination, candidates will not receive any feedback about their performance. However, all candidates will receive written notification of their results within 6 to 8 weeks after the examination. The ACSM cannot give examination results over the telephone.

CONTINUING EDUCATION CREDITS (CECS)

To ensure ongoing competency and to maintain a high standard for certified professionals, every ACSM-certified individual is reviewed on a 4-year basis. Continuing certification is granted to candidates who successfully:

1. Document the required ACSM Continuing Education Credits (CECs), ACSM Continuing Medical Education Credits (CMEs), or the equivalent, and
2. Maintain a current cardiopulmonary resuscitation (CPR) certification.

The total number of CECs required for each certification level for a 4-year period is as follows:

ACSM Health/Fitness Director®—120
ACSM Health/Fitness Instructor_SM—80
ACSM Exercise Leader®—40

CECs can be earned in the following ways:

1. Earning ACSM CECs/CMEs or credits from other qualified professional organizations by attending professional meetings or by taking continuing education self-tests, such as those found in professional journals.
2. Taking and receiving a passing grade in a course from an accredited college or university that maintains or enhances professional development.

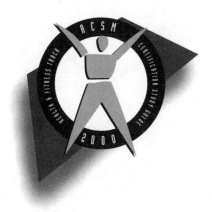

RESULTS AND RETESTS

The written and practical examinations are scored through the ACSM National Center. The results of the written and practical examinations are mailed directly to the candidate from the ACSM National Center approximately 6 to 8 weeks following an examination. Candidates pass or fail the practical examination as a total entity.

A candidate may be retested on the written examination, practical examination, or both, if necessary. Candidates who fail the written or practical examination must submit a retest application form with the accompanying retest fee to the ACSM National Center to be eligible to sit for the certification examination again. The minimum processing period for this retest application is 30 days. The application must be postmarked no later than 30 days prior to the start of the certification at the designated certification site that the candidate is choosing to attend. No application will be accepted after this date.

Candidates have 1 year from their original test date to successfully complete certification. There is no limit on the number of times the candidate can sit for the examination during the 1-year period as long as the above guidelines are followed.

CERTIFICATION RENEWAL

A certified professional who has gained certification at more than one level can choose which certification(s) to keep current. The documentation for currency at one level can be duplicated for the other levels of certification for the appropriate period.

The renewal fees for continuing certification are as follows:

ACSM Health/Fitness Director®—$80
ACSM Program Director$_{SM}$—$80
ACSM Health/Fitness Instructor$_{SM}$—$60
ACSM Exercise Specialist®—$60
ACSM Exercise Leader®—$60

A $5 fee is charged for all additional certifications that one wishes to keep current. For example, if one wishes to maintain both the ACSM Health/Fitness Director® and the ACSM Health/Fitness Instructor$_{SM}$ certifications, the renewal fees would be $85 ($80 for the ACSM Health/Fitness Director® and $5 for the additional ACSM Health/Fitness Instructor$_{SM}$ certification).

ACSM Exercise Leader® Certification

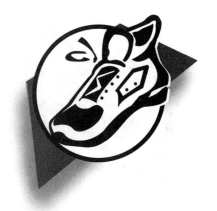

The ACSM Exercise Leader® is the professional involved in group exercise leadership. Using a variety of teaching techniques, the Exercise Leader is proficient in leading and demonstrating safe and effective methods of exercise by applying the fundamental principles of exercise science. The ACSM Exercise Leader® is familiar with all forms of group exercise including such as but not limited to traditional low, high, mixed, and step aerobics; slide, stationary indoor cycling, interval, circuit, water, muscle conditioning, yoga, and flexibility training. The following material will be helpful in preparing for both the written and practical examinations. All information should be read carefully.

MINIMUM REQUIREMENTS AND RECOMMENDED COMPETENCIES

Minimum Requirements

➤ Fitness certification from a nationally recognized organization

OR

➤ Completed or current enrollment in exercise-related college courses at a regionally accredited college/university

OR

➤ 300 hours of group exercise instruction experience

AND

➤ Possess current cardiopulmonary resuscitation (CPR) certification.

Recommended Competencies

1. Demonstrate practical skills and abilities associated with group exercise leadership.
2. Demonstrate the ability to positively motivate, communicate, and interact effectively with members of the group.
3. Possess adequate knowledge of how the body responds to, and is affected by, exercise.

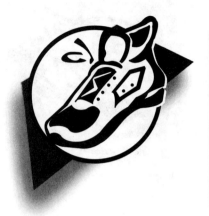

4. Demonstrate the ability to safely apply the principles of exercise and training to group fitness programs.

5. Demonstrate the ability to answer basic questions relating to exercise science and to refer others to appropriate sources of information.

6. Possess a basic knowledge of exercise science including kinesiology, functional anatomy, exercise physiology, group exercise programming, nutrition, and injury prevention.

WORKSHOP INFORMATION

At some sites, a workshop may be conducted before the ACSM Exercise Leader® certification. The Exercise Leader workshop is optional and is not a prerequisite for certification. The workshop is designed to develop and enhance the knowledge base and practical skills of the exercise leader. This way, the student is able to combine theory and practice.

All workshop participants should have an active interest in the health and fitness profession. There are no absolute prerequisites for the workshop. However, participants without knowledge and background in the health and fitness profession should understand that the workshop is not intended to provide the full experience and knowledge necessary for ACSM certification, as described in the KSAs in the Appendix of the 6th edition of *ACSM's Guidelines for Exercise Testing and Prescription*.

CERTIFICATION INFORMATION

The ACSM Exercise Leader® certification encompasses written and practical examination competencies. The candidate must successfully complete both written and practical components to receive ACSM certification. The two components are scored separately, and a passing score is required in each component.

Written Examination

The written examination contains approximately 100 multiple choice questions drawn from the KSAs in the Appendix of the 6th edition of *ACSM's Guidelines for Exercise Testing and Prescription*. KSAs outline minimal competencies necessary for certification. The table below lists the approximate number of questions from each of the areas represented by KSAs.

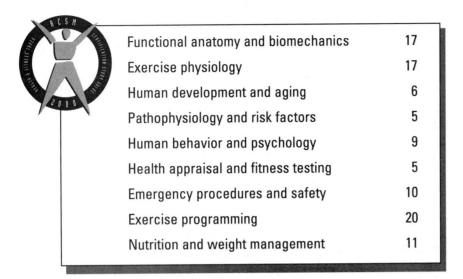

Functional anatomy and biomechanics	17
Exercise physiology	17
Human development and aging	6
Pathophysiology and risk factors	5
Human behavior and psychology	9
Health appraisal and fitness testing	5
Emergency procedures and safety	10
Exercise programming	20
Nutrition and weight management	11

Sample Questions/Answers

It is ACSM's goal to make this certification process a positive experience for all participants. Therefore, sample questions have been developed to help determine a candidate's current level of preparation. The following sample questions will help the candidate test his or her knowledge base in preparation for the written portion of the Exercise Leader examination. The answers follow the last question. Candidates are encouraged to review, in detail, those topics for which his or her answers were incorrect.

1. When doing a push-up, which phase is considered concentric for the triceps muscle group?
   a. Pressing up, so that the elbows straighten
   b. Lowering down, so that the elbows bend
   c. Both up and down are concentric
   d. Neither is concentric, this is an isometric exercise

2. An exaggerated curve in the lower back is referred to as:
   a. excessive kyphosis.
   b. scoliosis.
   c. excessive lordosis.
   d. low back pain syndrome.

3. The primary energy system used for the 100-meter dash is:
   a. aerobic glycolysis.
   b. anaerobic glycolysis.
   c. Kreb's cycle.
   d. ATP-CP system.

4. An increase in submaximal exercise intensity will result in:
   a. an increase in systolic and diastolic blood pressure.
   b. a decrease in systolic and diastolic blood pressure.
   c. an increase in systolic blood pressure as diastolic stays the same or decreases.
   d. an increase in diastolic blood pressure as systolic stays the same or decreases.

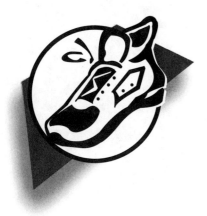

5. Each of the following is a sign of overtraining **except:**

   a. performance decrements.
   b. mood disturbance.
   c. decreased resting heart rate.
   d. elevated resting blood pressure.

6. John Smith is 43. His blood pressure is 128/82 mm Hg, and his cholesterol level is 222 mg/dL. He has a very stressful job and has not exercised in 7 years. John's 70-year-old mother had a heart attack last year. According to the ACSM, how many positive coronary artery disease risk factors does John have?

   a. Five
   b. Four
   c. Three
   d. Two

7. All of the following muscles are in the hamstring group **except:**

   a. rectus femoris.
   b. semimembranosus.
   c. biceps femoris.
   d. semitendinosus.

8. Stressing a physiological system slightly beyond what it is accustomed to is called:

   a. specificity.
   b. reversibility.
   c. overload.
   d. plyometrics.

9. Individuals with excessive lordosis should:

   a. strengthen abdominals and stretch hip flexors and erector spinae.
   b. strengthen hip flexors and stretch abdominals.
   c. increase the amount of cardiorespiratory exercise.
   d. avoid exercise.

10. Which of the following is the **least** accurate way to assess body composition?

    a. Height and weight charts
    b. Bioelectrical impedance
    c. Skinfolds
    d. Hydrostatic weighing

11. Which of the following responses would you typically observe if an initially sedentary person completed 20 weeks of regular cardiorespiratory conditioning?

    a. Lower resting stroke volume, higher resting heart rate
    b. Lower resting stroke volume, lower resting heart rate
    c. Higher resting stroke volume, higher resting heart rate
    d. Higher resting stroke volume, lower resting heart rate

12. Which of the following is a fat-soluble vitamin?

    a. Vitamin A
    b. Vitamin C
    c. Vitamin B complex
    d. None of the above

13. Which of the following types of resistance training programs is considered static?
    a. Isometric
    b. Isotonic
    c. Circuit
    d. Pyramid

14. A hurdler's stretch may place inappropriate stress on which of the following areas?
    a. Ankle
    b. Knee
    c. Hip
    d. Back

15. A food label states that 10 g of carbohydrate and 4 g of fat are contained in one serving. Calculate the total kcal of carbohydrate and fat.
    a. 90 kcal carbohydrate; 16 kcal fat
    b. 60 kcal carbohydrate; 40 kcal fat
    c. 40 kcal carbohydrate; 36 kcal fat
    d. 80 kcal carbohydrate; 20 kcal fat

16. Frank is 50 years old and has a resting heart rate of 60 beats/minute (bpm). Using the Karvonen formula, calculate his target heart rate range if he would like to exercise at 60–70% of his age-predicted maximum heart rate.
    a. 126–137 bpm
    b. 137–148 bpm
    c. 115–126 bpm
    d. 130–141 bpm

17. The component of an exercise prescription that plays the most important role in preventing blood pooling is:
    a. warm-up.
    b. stimulus-aerobic conditioning.
    c. muscular strength training.
    d. cool-down.

18. All of the following are considered a benefit of regular physical activity **except:**
    a. increased serum high-density lipoprotein (HDL) cholesterol.
    b. lower heart rate and blood pressure at a given submaximal intensity.
    c. enhanced feelings of well-being.
    d. increased insulin needs with a decrease in glucose tolerance.

19. After the first trimester, pregnant women should avoid exercise in which of the following positions?
    a. Lying on the left side
    b. Lying on the right side
    c. Supine
    d. Hands and knees

20. Examples of overuse injuries include all of the following **except:**
    a. compound fractures.
    b. shin splints.
    c. tendonitis.
    d. stress fractures.

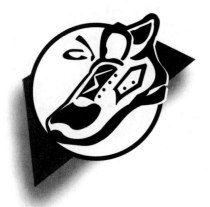

21. What neural receptors are responsible for initiating the stretch reflex?

   a. Golgi spindle
   b. Muscle spindle
   c. Motor end plates
   d. Muscle fibers

22. The vastus lateralis:

   a. flexes the knee.
   b. flexes the foot.
   c. extends the knee.
   d. extends the hip.

23. To effectively monitor intensity during a 25-minute cardiorespiratory workout, the heart rate and/or rating of perceived exertion (RPE) should be measured:

   a. at the end of the cardiorespiratory segment.
   b. at the beginning of the cardiorespiratory segment.
   c. after at least 3 to 5 minutes of cardiorespiratory exercise.
   d. after 1 to 2 minutes of cardiorespiratory exercise.

24. According to the American College of Obstetricians and Gynecologists guidelines for exercise during pregnancy and postpartum:

   a. intermittent exercise is preferred over exercising regularly 3 times a week.
   b. women who exercise in the first trimester should ensure adequate hydration.
   c. women should avoid exercise in the supine position throughout their entire pregnancy.
   d. many of the physiological changes with pregnancy subside immediately after delivery.

25. In most aerobic exercise activities, heart rate has a linear relationship with:

   a. $\dot{V}O_2$.
   b. rating of perceived exertion (RPE).
   c. age.
   d. weight.

Answers

1. a	**8.** c	**15.** c	**22.** c
2. c	**9.** a	**16.** a	**23.** c
3. d	**10.** a	**17.** d	**24.** b
4. c	**11.** d	**18.** d	**25.** a
5. c	**12.** a	**19.** c	
6. d	**13.** a	**20.** a	
7. a	**14.** b	**21.** b	

Practical Examination

The practical examination is composed of three separate test stations, each 20 minutes in length, for a total of 60 minutes. Time limitations are strictly enforced to ensure equity among candidates. The candidate must attain an overall passing score for successful completion of the practical examination. Each station has an objective checklist of skills and/or actions on which the examiner documents the results. The practical examination is then scored through the ACSM National Center. As with the written examination, competencies are based on the KSAs.

Before the written and practical examinations, the Certification Director will conduct a candidate meeting to answer questions concerning the certification process. In addition, all certification candidates will have the opportunity to review the equipment that will be used. There will be no instruction provided. This review period is typically scheduled the afternoon or evening before the practical examination. The Site Director or Certification Director at the testing site will provide the time schedule for review. The Certification Director will also be responsible for administering the certification evaluation at the completion of the certification exam. Candidates are encouraged to provide feedback concerning the certification process; however, no discussion of examination content will occur at this time.

Practical Examination Stations

Station 1. Group Leadership: Warm-up, Cardiorespiratory Stimulus, Post-cardiorespiratory Cool-down.

The candidate will demonstrate the ability to:

> A. Teach an effective warm-up that will prepare a group of apparently healthy adults for cardiorespiratory exercise.
> B. Teach a group of apparently healthy adults an appropriate cardiorespiratory stimulus using high- and/or low-impact aerobic movements or step exercise followed by a post-cardiorespiratory cool-down.
> C. Demonstrate and cue proper exercise technique and body alignment. Communicate and interact effectively with the group and with individual members of the group.

Time allotments for this session are as follows:

Warm-up: 4 to 6 minutes
Cardiorespiratory stimulus: 5 to 7 minutes
Post-cardiorespiratory cool-down: 2 to 4 minutes

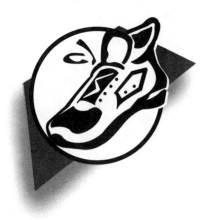

Note: The candidate may choose to use music for this station. The music must be appropriate in terms of pace and volume and should complement the routine. A cassette player will be available; however, sites will not provide music.

■ SOURCES

ACSM. *ACSM's Guidelines for Exercise Testing and Prescription.* 6th ed. Baltimore: Lippincott Williams & Wilkins, 2000.

ACSM. *ACSM's Resource Manual for Guidelines for Exercise Testing and Prescription.* 3rd ed. Baltimore: Williams & Wilkins, 1998.

Aerobics and Fitness Association of America. *Fitness: Theory & Practice.* 2nd ed. Sherman Oaks, CA: Aerobics and Fitness Association of America, 1995.

Aerobics and Fitness Association of America. *Step Training: A Manual for Instructors.* Sherman Oaks, CA: Aerobics and Fitness Association of America, 1997.

Cotton R, ed. *Aerobics Instructor Manual: The Resource of Fitness Professionals.* San Diego, CA: American Council on Exercise, 1993.

Kennedy C, Legel D. *Anatomy of an Exercise Class: An Exercise Educator's Handbook.* Champaign, IL: Sagamore Publishing, 1992.

Stanforth D, Ellison D. *Aerobic Dance Exercise.* St. Louis: Mosby-Year Book, 1997.

Station 2. Group Leadership: Muscle Conditioning

The candidate will demonstrate the ability to:

A. Teach safe, effective, and appropriate muscle conditioning exercises in the group setting.

B. Modify muscle conditioning exercises as necessary to accommodate the needs of the following special populations: pregnant, elderly, obese, low back discomfort, and novice.

C. Demonstrate and cue proper exercise technique and body alignment.

D. Communicate and interact effectively with the group and with individual members of the group.

■ SOURCES

ACSM. *ACSM's Guidelines for Exercise Testing and Prescription.* 6th ed. Baltimore: Lippincott Williams & Wilkins, 2000.

Aerobics and Fitness Association of America. *Fitness: Theory & Practice.* 2nd ed. Sherman Oaks, CA: Aerobics and Fitness Association of America, 1995.

Baechle TR, Groves BR. *Essentials of Strength Training and Conditioning.* Champaign, IL: Human Kinetics, 1994.

Cailliet R. *Understand Your Backache.* Philadelphia: FA Davis, 1987.

Cotton R, ed. *Aerobics Instructor Manual: The Resource of Fitness Professionals.* San Diego, CA: American Council on Exercise, 1993.
Kennedy C, Legel D. *Anatomy of an Exercise Class: An Exercise Educator's Handbook.* Champaign, IL: Sagamore Publishing, 1992.
Noble E. *Essential Exercises for the Childbearing Years.* 3rd ed. Boston: Houghton Mifflin, 1998.

Station 3. Group Leadership: Flexibility

The candidate will demonstrate the ability to:

A. Teach safe, effective, and appropriate flexibility exercises in the group setting.

B. Modify flexibility exercises as necessary to accommodate the needs of the following special populations: pregnant, elderly, obese, low back discomfort, and novice.

C. Demonstrate and cue proper exercise technique and body alignment.

D. Communicate and interact effectively with the group and with individual members of the group.

■ **SOURCES**

ACSM. *ACSM's Guidelines for Exercise Testing and Prescription.* 6th ed. Baltimore: Lippincott Williams & Wilkins, 2000.
ACSM. *ACSM's Resource Manual for Guidelines for Exercise Testing and Prescription.* 3rd ed. Baltimore: Williams & Wilkins, 1998.
Aerobics and Fitness Association of America. *Fitness: Theory & Practice.* 2nd ed. Sherman Oaks, CA: Aerobics and Fitness Association of America, 1995.
Alter MJ. *Science of Flexibility.* 2nd ed. Champaign, IL: Human Kinetics, 1996.
Cotton R, ed. *Aerobics Instructor Manual: The Resource of Fitness Professionals.* San Diego, CA: American Council on Exercise, 1993.
Franks BD, Howley ET. *Fitness Leader's Handbook.* Champaign, IL: Human Kinetics, 1989.
Noble E. *Essential Exercises for the Childbearing Years.* 3rd ed. Boston: Houghton Mifflin, 1998.

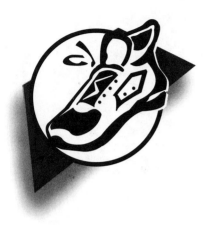

CERTIFICATION CONTENT MATERIAL

Coronary Artery Disease Risk Factors

Coronary artery disease (CAD) is the single leading cause of premature death in the United States. It is estimated that CAD is responsible for more than 48% of all deaths and that 1 of every 5 people whose death is attributable to CAD is younger than 65. In many cases, premature death and disability from CAD can be prevented. Epidemiologic studies have found that several characteristics are highly related to the development of CAD, and these are referred to as risk factors. Although some risk factors (age, family history) cannot be altered by modifying lifestyle behaviors, others (hypertension, smoking, hypercholesterolemia, non–insulin-dependent diabetes mellitus [NIDDM], physical inactivity) can be favorably altered with healthy habits.

Positive Risk Factors	Defining Criteria
1. Age	Men older than 45; women older than 55 or who experience premature menopause without estrogen replacement therapy.
2. Family history	Myocardial infarction or sudden death before 55 years of age in father or other male, first-degree relative. Myocardial infarction or sudden death before 65 years of age in mother or other female, first-degree relative.
3. Current cigarette smoking	
4. Hypertension	Blood pressure > 140/90 mm Hg, confirmed by measurements on at least two separate occasions, or taking antihypertensive medication.
5. Hypercholesterolemia	Total serum cholesterol > 200 mg/dL (5.2 mmol/L) (if lipoprotein profile is unavailable) or high-density lipoprotein (HDL) < 35 mg/dL (0.9 mmol/L).
6. Diabetes mellitus	Persons with insulin-dependent diabetes mellitus (IDDM) who are older than 30 or have had IDDM for more than 15 years and persons with NIDDM who are older than 35 should be classified as patients with disease.
7. Sedentary lifestyle	Persons comprising the least active 25% of the population as defined by the combination of sedentary jobs involving sitting for a large part of the day and no regular exercise or active recreational pursuits.

Negative Risk Factor	Comment
1. High serum HDL cholesterol	>60 mg/dL (1.6 mmol/L)

Notes: (1) It is common to sum risk factors in making clinical judgments. If HDL is high, subtract one risk factor from the sum of positive risk factors, because high HDL decreases CAD risk. (2) Obesity is not listed as an independent positive risk factor because its effects are exerted through other risk factors (e.g., hypertension, hyperlipidemia, diabetes). Obesity should be considered as an independent target for intervention.

Hypertension is a chronic, persistent elevation of blood pressure that affects an estimated one of every four adults in the United States. A sodium-restricted diet, weight reduction, restricted alcohol intake, and exercise may help to lower blood pressure. Additionally, many antihypertensive drugs are available to lower blood pressure.

Hypercholesterolemia is an elevation in blood cholesterol. In the body, cholesterol is transported as lipoproteins, a lipid bound to a protein carrier. Low-density lipoproteins (LDLs) are large molecules that are actively transported into the vascular walls. LDLs stimulate the formation of plaque, which reduces the cross-sectional area of the blood vessels and obstructs blood flow. An obstruction in the coronary arteries may produce a myocardial infarction. HDLs are smaller molecules and serve a protective function by picking up excess cholesterol from arterial walls and removing it from the body.

Cigarette smokers have more than twice the risk of heart attack as nonsmokers. The nicotine contained in cigarette smoke produces an increase in blood pressure and heart rate and inhibits the anti-clotting mechanisms of the blood. When an individual stops smoking, the risk of CAD declines rapidly. According to the American Heart Association, the risk of death from CAD for individuals who had smoked a pack a day or less and who have since quit is almost the same as that of persons who never smoked.

Diabetes mellitus is characterized by a chronically elevated blood glucose concentration. Insulin-dependent diabetes mellitus (IDDM or type 1) results from a deficiency in insulin production. Persons with IDDM are usually dependent on regular injections of insulin, usually given at least twice per day. Non–insulin-dependent diabetes mellitus (NIDDM or type 2) is usually associated with decreased cellular insulin sensitivity. Approximately 90% of all diabetics have NIDDM, which is linked to obesity. The primary treatment of persons with NIDDM includes diet and exercise to reduce body weight and to help control blood glucose.

Several epidemiologic studies have demonstrated that more active individuals have a lower risk of heart disease than sedentary individuals. Recent studies indicate that both physical activity, such as expending more than 2000 kcal/week in physical activity, and car-

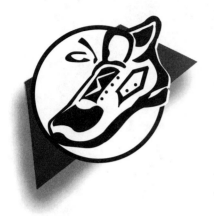

diovascular fitness levels are major factors related to the prevention of CAD. Additionally, regular exercise may modify other CAD risk factors by improving serum cholesterol levels, decreasing blood pressure, and improving glucose tolerance.

Initial Risk Stratification

1. Apparently healthy: individuals who are asymptomatic and apparently healthy with no more than one major coronary risk factor.
2. Increased risk: individuals who have signs or symptoms suggestive of possible cardiopulmonary or metabolic disease and/or two or more major coronary risk factors.
3. Known disease: individuals with known cardiac, pulmonary, or metabolic disease.

Anatomy and Kinesiology

Directional Terminology

Anatomic position: position of the body when the subject is facing front in the erect position with the arms and legs fully extended. The palms of the hands are facing forward, and the feet are together. This term is used as the reference position of the body to describe various positions.

Supine position: position in which the subject is lying on the back with the face up.

Prone position: position in which the subject is lying on the front of the body with the face down.

Anterior: in front of.

Posterior: in back of.

Medial: toward the midline of the body.

Lateral: away from the midline of the body.

Proximal: closer to the point of attachment or origin; in the extremities, closest to the trunk.

Distal: farther from the point of attachment or origin; in the extremities, farthest from the trunk.

Superior: toward the head, above.

Inferior: away from the head, below.

Superficial: toward the surface of the body.

Deep: inside the body and away from the body surface.

Movement Terminology

Flexion: decreasing the joint angle between two bones, as in bending the elbow or knee. Most flexion movements are forward movements; a major exception is flexion of the knee.

Extension: increasing the joint angle between two bones and returning toward the anatomic position, as in straightening the knee or elbow. Most extension movements are backward movements; a major exception is the extension of the knee.

Hyperextension: movement of any joint beyond the joint's normal position of extension (during a swan dive, the cervical and lumbar spine are in hyperextension).

Abduction: movement away from the midline of the body (raising the arms out to the side).

Adduction: moving toward the midline of the body (returning laterally raised arms to the side of the body).

Rotation: movement of a long bone clockwise or counterclockwise around its long axis. Rotation toward midline is medial (internal) rotation and away from the midline is lateral (external) rotation.

Circumduction: a circular movement around a joint (movement in 360°); the swing of a limb whose distal end forms a circle and whose proximal end forms the apex (tip) of the cone (combination of flexion, extension, abduction, and adduction movements).

Specialized Movement Terminology

Lateral flexion: sideways tilt of the head or trunk.

Scapular elevation: raising the scapula, as in a shoulder shrug.

Scapular depression: lowering motion of the scapula.

Scapular abduction (protraction): scapulae move away from each other, as occurs when rounding the shoulders.

Scapular adduction (retraction): scapulae move toward each other with the shoulders back.

Scapular upward rotation: scapulae swing out, so that the bottom of the scapulae move away from midline of body and the top of the scapulae move toward the midline.

Scapular downward rotation: scapulae swing back down to resting position.

Horizontal-adduction (-flexion): movement at shoulder of bringing upper arm toward the midline in the horizontal plane (moving arms that are raised out to the side toward the front of the body).

Horizontal-abduction (-extension): movement at shoulder of bringing upper arm away from the midline in the horizontal plane.

Supination: moving forearm palms down to palms up.

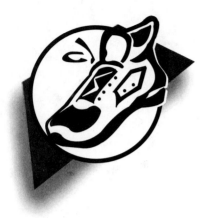

Pronation: moving forearm palms up to palms down.

Plantar flexion: extending (planting) the ankle, increasing the angle between the dorsal (top) part of the foot and the anterior tibia (angle between the foot and leg increases); pointing the toe.

Dorsiflexion: flexing the ankle so that the angle between the dorsal (top) part of the foot and anterior tibia decreases (angle between the leg and foot decreases); point toes toward head.

Inversion: moving the ankle laterally outward so that the sole of the foot points toward the midline (soles of the feet pointing toward each other).

Eversion: moving the ankle medially inward so that the sole of the foot points away from the midline (soles of feet point away from each other).

Types of Planes

Planes geometrically bisect the body and describe bodily movements. Movements take place alongside of or next to the planes.

Horizontal plane (transverse): divides the body into upper and lower portions.

Frontal plane (coronal): divides the body into front and back.

Sagittal plane (medial): divides the body into right and left portions.

Types of Joints

Type	Movement	Example
Hinge	Flexion and extension on one axis	Knee, elbow, finger (between phalanges)
Ellipsoidal (condyloid)	Flexion, extension, abduction, adduction (biaxial)	Wrist (radius with carpals) Knuckle (metacarpal with phalange)
Gliding plane	Slipping or gliding	Intercarpal (one carpal bone moving over another carpal bone)
Pivot	Rotation	Radius and distal end of humerus
Ball and socket	All movements (flexion, extension, abduction, adduction, and rotation)	Hip, shoulder
Saddle	All movements plus opposition	Carpal bone (trapezium and first metacarpal)

Joint Actions and Prime Movers

Shoulder

Flexion:
  Pectoralis major, clavicular
  Anterior deltoid

Extension:
  Latissimus dorsi
  Teres major
  Pectoralis major, sternal

Abduction:
  Medial deltoid
  Supraspinatus

Adduction:
  Latissimus dorsi
  Teres major
  Pectoralis major, sternal

Horizontal abduction:
  Posterior deltoid
  Infraspinatus
  Teres minor

Horizontal adduction:
  Pectoralis major, clavicular
    and sternal
  Anterior deltoid
  Coracobrachialis

Internal rotation:
  Subscapularis
  Teres major

External rotation:
  Infraspinatus
  Teres minor

Shoulder Girdle

Scapular elevation:
  Trapezius, upper
  Rhomboids
  Levator scapulae

Scapular adduction (retraction):
  Trapezius, middle
  Rhomboids

Scapular upward rotation:
  Serratus anterior
  Trapezius, upper and lower

Scapular depression:
  Trapezius, lower
  Pectoralis minor

Scapular abduction (protraction):
  Serratus anterior
  Pectoralis minor

Scapular downward rotation:
  Rhomboids
  Pectoralis minor

Elbow

Flexion:
  Biceps brachii
  Brachialis
  Brachioradialis

Extension:
  Triceps brachii
  Anconeus

Spine

Flexion:
  Rectus abdominis
  Internal/external obliques

Extension:
  Erector spinae

Lateral flexion:
  Quadratus lumborum
  Internal/external obliques

Spinal rotation:
  Internal/external obliques

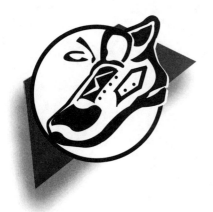

Hip

Flexion:
  Iliacus
  Psoas
  Rectus femoris
  Pectineus

Extension:
  Biceps femoris
  Semimembranosus
  Semitendinosus
  Gluteus maximus

Adduction:
  Adductor magnus
  Adductor brevis
  Adductor longus
  Gracilis
  Pectineus

Abduction:
  Gluteus medius
  Tensor fascia latae

Inward rotation:
  Gluteus minimus

Outward rotation:
  Gluteus maximus
  Piriformis
  Quadratus femoris
  Gemellus superior
  Gemellus inferior
  Obturator internus
  Obturator externus

Knee

Extension:
Rectus femoris
Vastus lateralis
Vastus medialis
Vastus intermedius

Flexion:
Biceps femoris
Semitendinosus
Semimembranosus

Ankle

Dorsiflexion:
Tibialis anterior
Peroneus tertius
Extensor digitorum
  longus

Plantar flexion:
Gastrocnemius
Soleus

Inversion:
Anterior tibialis
Posterior tibialis

Eversion:
Extensor digitorum longus
Peroneus tertius
Peroneus longus
Peroneus brevis

Heart Rate Measurement

Heart rate is the number of beats the heart makes per minute. Resting heart rate and heart rate during a standard submaximal workload are useful indicators of cardiorespiratory fitness levels because both decrease as an individual becomes more fit. Exercise heart rate can be useful in monitoring the intensity of exercise. Generally, the higher the workload, the higher the heart rate response, thus the higher the intensity of the exercise. Because there is a linear relationship between heart rate and workload in aerobic exercise, one can estimate maximal oxygen consumption ($\dot{V}O_{2max}$). This information is used to give the participant feedback regarding level of fitness. The higher the maximal oxygen consumption, the higher the cardiorespiratory fitness level.

Similar increases in cardiorespiratory endurance may be achieved by a low-intensity, long-duration training program as by a high-intensity, shorter-duration training program. High-intensity programs are not appropriate for sedentary individuals due to an increased risk of injury. Most individuals begin with a lower intensity, longer duration program. In fact, studies indicate that individuals who participate in exercise intensities that are inappropriately high, demonstrate lower adherence to exercise versus individuals who exercise at a more appropriate lower intensity.

Resting heart rate alone is not an indicator of fitness, although resting heart rate tends to decline over time with appropriate training. With appropriate frequency, intensity, and duration, the heart muscle becomes a stronger, more efficient pump. Therefore, it performs the same amount of work with fewer beats.

Maximal heart rate is not affected by training, but decreases with age. The 1998 ACSM Position Stand on Quantity and Quality of Exercise for Healthy Adults states that appropriate exercise intensity falls within 55 to 90% of age-predicted maximal heart rate, where maximal heart rate is determined by subtracting age from 220. Exercise intensity can also be expressed as a percentage of heart rate reserve. The Position Stand states that 40 to 85% of heart rate reserve (Karvonen formula) may also be appropriate for determining appropriate exercise intensity. The lower intensity values (i.e., 55 to 64% of age-predicted maximum heart rate) and 40 to 49% of heart rate reserve (HRR) are most applicable to individuals who are deconditioned (American College of Sports Medicine Position Stand. The recommended quantity and quality of exercise for developing and maintaining cardiovascular and muscular fitness, and flexibility in healthy adults. *Med Sci Sports Exerc* 1998;30:975–991).

Resting and exercise heart rate can be measured by palpating the pulse at one of two sites (see Palpation below). Resting heart rate can be counted for 10, 15, 30, or 60 seconds, with the 30- and 60-second counts being the most accurate. During steady-state exercise, for best accuracy, it is recommended that heart rates be counted for 10 seconds. The shorter times are used when the heart rate recovers (slows down) during counting. The 10-second count should be multiplied by 6 in order to calculate the heart rate in beats per minute (bpm). Heart rate should not be measured until at least 3 to 5 minutes into exercise in order to allow the heart rate to achieve steady state.

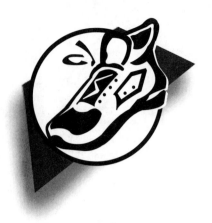

Palpation

1. Most common sites:

   Radial artery: on the anterolateral aspect of the wrist directly in line with the base of the thumb.

   Carotid artery: in the neck, just lateral to the larynx.

2. The tip of the middle and index fingers should be used. The thumb should not be used because it has a pulse of its own and may produce an inaccurate count.

3. When palpating the carotid site, light pressure should be used. Baroreceptors in the carotid arteries detect heavy pressure and cause a reflex slowing of the heart.

4. The number of beats should be counted for the designated period.

Group Exercise Leadership

Basics of Leadership

Effective group leadership is associated with a variety of personal skills and characteristics. These skills include such factors as professional appearance, organization of activities, communication, motivation, individual attention and feedback, safety monitoring, and the ability to demonstrate exercise with appropriate form and alignment.

An effective group exercise leader does not necessarily have to be the most fit and most energetic person in the group. However, a professional demeanor and respect for group members as participants who are seeking positive experiences with physical activity and exercise are paramount. The group leader should wear attire that is not intimidating, appeals to various types of participants, is appropriate for the type of class, and conveys a professional image.

It is very important that group exercise leaders have the ability to demonstrate a variety of movements and exercises with appropriate form and technique. Participants in group exercise tend to rely heavily on visual sense and often unconsciously copy the instructor's alignment and technique. Skill in demonstration and the maintenance of good alignment on the part of the exercise leader makes it more likely that the participant will exercise safely and effectively. However, there are effective leaders who may not be able to demonstrate appropriate technique, but who are able to use verbal cues and hands-on correction to assist participants in achieving the correct form and alignment. Exercise leaders should be able to stabilize the spine, pelvis, and scapulae while performing exercises for the extremities in a variety of positions (standing, bent over, seated, side-lying, all fours, supine, prone) and should be able to demonstrate correct form while lifting.

Teaching and leadership styles are influenced by many factors including individual participant characteristics (age, skill, fitness level), class size, time allotted per class, time of day for class, availability of aides, equipment, and facilities. A successful group exercise leader must have effective organizational skills. Leaders should be aware of a variety of organizational patterns to provide clear observation of their participants.

Oral communication skills are essential to quality group leadership. Leaders should understand the various aspects of communication including content, verbal and nonverbal delivery, and how the participant receives the message. Leaders should strive to develop communication skills in order to interact more effectively with the group and with individual members of the group.

Effective cueing is one way to enhance communication. Several types of cues should be used during the exercise session:

Anticipatory cues: Cues that let participants know what moves are next so that the group moves smoothly and safely.

Informational and educational cues: These cues teach participants about their muscles, cardiorespiratory system, components of fitness, and wellness strategies.

Safety and alignment cues: These are important to ensure safety and effectiveness of the movements. Participants are instructed how to stabilize/move various joints and about the risks of incorrect technique.

Motivational cues: Cues that give general and specific praise. This helps increase positive energy and a sense of fun. These types of cues should be used frequently!

The ability to create a positive atmosphere and to positively motivate the members of the group is another important trait necessary for effective group leadership. One way to motivate is to educate. The group exercise leader has a unique opportunity to provide educational experiences for the group members by addressing a variety of issues ranging from exercise techniques to monitoring exercise intensity. One of the most important educational responsibilities of the group leader is to teach the responsibility for self. In other words, each participant should be exposed to information about basic exercise principles in order to ensure a safe and effective workout in a variety of exercise settings. Teaching participants how to monitor exercise heart rate and how to use the Rating of Perceived Exertion (RPE) chart is an example of teaching self-responsibility. The group exercise leader must be able to make fitness fun and enjoyable and must be able to disseminate accurate information.

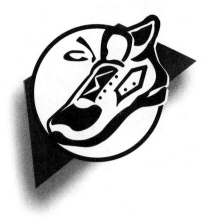

Basic Structure of a Group Exercise Session

Warm-up Phase

The objectives of the warm-up include increasing the heart rate and joint range of motion. The first component of the warm-up comprises movements involving large muscle groups. This dynamic phase results in an increased heart rate and an elevated muscle temperature, which produces an increase in the elastic property of the muscles. This improvement in the elastic property of the muscle allows for more effective stretching, which is the second component of the warm-up. Stretching during warm-up may play a role in reducing the risk of injury and in reducing the symptoms of muscle soreness.

Static stretching is performed to prepare muscles for exercise, by moving them, at least once, through a full range of motion prior to vigorous activity. Since the purpose of static stretching in the warm-up is not the enhancement of flexibility, a shorter duration of approximately 10 seconds is acceptable.

Ballistic stretches should be discouraged for most participants because they increase the risk of injury. Some commonly used stretching exercises may not be appropriate for many participants; these include straight-leg standing toe touches, the yoga plow, 360° head rolls, full squats, swan back stretch, hurdler's stretch, and shoulder stands. Care should be taken to provide modifications for stretches that could compromise the safety of any member of the group.

The following general recommendations should be used for proper warm-up activities:

➤ Both dynamic and static components should be included in the warm-up.
➤ The participant should start slowly and gradually increase intensity and range of motion.
➤ The intensity and length of the warm-up should stimulate an increased breathing rate, increased heart rate and light sweat; usually 5 to 10 minutes is an adequate length of time for warm-up.
➤ Muscles that will be used in the cardiorespiratory stimulus should be targeted in the warm-up.

Cardiorespiratory Stimulus Phase

The cardiorespiratory stimulus phase of the group exercise session may use a variety of modes and formats, including traditional high- and low-impact movements, step aerobics, combination classes, interval classes, slide, stationary indoor cycling, water aerobics, water jogging, stationary indoor rowing, walking, boxing, and other sports-specific modalities. Exercise intensity should be increased gradually, and participants should be instructed how to select the appropriate intensity for steady-state exercise. A variety of movements should be used to minimize excessive musculoskeletal stress and keep the workout fun and motivating. The stimulus phase should last 20 to 60 minutes.

The following general recommendations are suggested for providing a safe and enjoyable experience for participants:

➤ Gradually increase and decrease exercise intensity at the beginning and end of this segment.

➤ Maintain intensity while incorporating a variety of movements through full range of motion with proper form.

➤ Use a variety of large muscle groups.

➤ Promote independence and responsibility for self by choosing movements that build participant success.

➤ Minimize repetitive movements and emphasize fun and enthusiasm.

➤ Include an exercise intensity check (heart rate and/or RPE).

➤ Provide modifications based on heart rate/RPE results and encourage participants to work at individual levels and abilities.

Post-cardiorespiratory Cool-down Phase

All moderate or vigorous physical activity should be followed by a cool-down period, to allow the body to gradually return to the preexercise or postwarm-up state. Like warm-up, the cool-down is often performed too quickly or not at all. An effective cardiorespiratory cool-down lasts from 3 to 5 minutes and may be followed by static stretching of the muscle groups that were primarily challenged. The movements used in the warm-up can be used in the cool-down. Gradual reductions in activity level allow circulatory parameters, such as heart rate, to return to preexercise levels. An active cool-down (walking, marching in place, slow jogging) also helps to prevent blood pooling in the lower body. Blood pooling is a condition in which blood collects in the large veins of the legs. Blood pooling may occur if exercise is stopped abruptly or if the individual sits down immediately after exercise. This can cause the participant to become dizzy and/or faint.

Following the post-cardiorespiratory cool-down period, it is important to stretch the large muscle groups used during the cardiorespiratory stimulus. Some of the muscles that are commonly

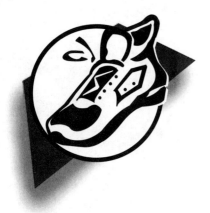

tight and should be addressed are the calves, hamstrings, low back, and hip flexors. The following general recommendations should be used for proper cool-down activities:

➤ The post-cardiorespiratory cool-down should be of sufficient length to allow for the postwarm-up heart rates to be achieved. One rule is to continue with the cool-down activities until the heart rates approach 100 bpm or lower.

➤ The post-cardiorespiratory cool-down should incorporate static stretches for the large muscle groups.

Muscle Conditioning

This phase of the exercise session incorporates activities that promote muscular strength and endurance. Balance and stability exercises may be included as well. Overload can be achieved by using different types of exercise equipment and by using a variety of positions such as standing, seated, side-lying, prone, supine, or on all fours. Resistance bands, hand-held weights, tubing, stability balls, bars, and body weight may be used to provide appropriate musculoskeletal resistance. The principle of overload is applied by increasing the amount of resistance and the number of repetitions and/or by progressing from easier to harder exercises. Safe and effective exercises should challenge the major muscle groups and promote muscle balance. Modifications should be provided for special populations such as pregnant women, the obese, people with a low back condition, and the elderly.

The following movements may not be appropriate for the group exercise setting: straight-leg sit-ups, double leg lifts, arched back push-ups, donkey kicks, arched trunk rolls, and deep knee bends. Any exercise should be modified, or an alternative sought, if the majority of the participants have difficulty maintaining proper alignment.

The following recommendations help provide a safe and effective experience for participants:

➤ Provide appropriate verbal cues on posture and alignment.

➤ Demonstrate proper body mechanics.

➤ Observe technique and form and adapt exercise for special populations.

➤ Correct and recommend changes in a polite, nonthreatening way.

➤ Use equipment safely and effectively.

Flexibility Phase

The end of every group exercise session should include a segment on flexibility. Cool-down stretches should focus on the large muscle groups used during the cardiorespiratory and muscle conditioning phases. Stretches are held approximately 15 to 30 seconds with the goal of muscle relaxation and maintaining or improving range of motion. Floor stretches are most common and minimize the effects of gravity. As in muscle conditioning, a variety of positions may be used and appropriate modifications for special populations should be provided.

The following general recommendations are suggested to enhance flexibility:

➤ Perform static stretches, holding each stretch for 15 to 30 seconds.

➤ Provide appropriate cueing while emphasizing relaxation.

➤ Stretch major muscle groups, especially those that are commonly tight, including the hamstrings, calves, hip flexors, low back, and chest.

Exercise Modifications for Special Populations

The following information provides basic recommendations and should not be viewed as a comprehensive description of an exercise prescription. For more complete information, refer to the references at the end of each certification section of this study guide.

Recommendations for Special Populations

	Exercise Prescription	Exercise Precautions
Hypertension	Frequency: 4–5 times/week Duration: 30–60 min Intensity: 40–70% $\dot{V}O_{2max}$ High-intensity and isometric activities should be avoided. Weight training should involve low resistance with high repetitions.	Medications may decrease training heart rate (THR). Longer cool-down. Medications limiting cardiac output: use RPE as an adjunct to HR. Diuretics may cause a decrease in K^+, leading to arrhythmias. Avoid Valsalva maneuvers.
Obesity	Goal: increase caloric expenditure. First choice: walking. Alternative modes: stair climbing, cycling, water exercise.	Avoid stress on joints. Choose setting that minimizes social stigma. Monitor muscle soreness and orthopedic problems.

continued

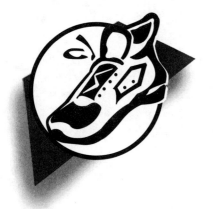

	Exercise Prescription	**Exercise Precautions**
Obesity, cont'd	Intensity at low end of target heart rate range. Duration sufficient to cause expenditure of 200–300 kcal.	Transition from standing to the floor and back to standing may be difficult. Supine abdominal and balance exercises may be difficult.
Diabetes	Daily exercise for IDDM; duration of 20–30 min/session achieve glucose control. NIDDM: maximize caloric expenditure if obese. May need to use RPE as adjunct to HR for monitoring exercise intensity.	Monitor blood glucose before and after exercise, especially when beginning a program. Adjustments in carbohydrate intake and/or insulin may be needed. Participant should measure blood glucose just prior to the exercise period and correct if too high or low. Attention to proper shoes and foot care. Understand what to do if the participant becomes hypoglycemic or hyperglycemic.
Children	Goal: increase energy expenditure, with minimal concern for exercise intensity emphasizing fun. Activities that require moving of whole body mass (walking, running, cycling, swimming) performed at lower intensity and longer duration. Body weight exercises for strength and muscle endurance.	Greater fatigability in prolonged high-intensity activities. Greater risk of heat-related illness. Higher incidence of overuse injuries. Use of weights, especially heavy weights, may place excessive stress on growth plates.
Low back	Goal: increase flexibility/ROM; aerobic conditioning; strength and endurance of the trunk and lower body. Support of back with sitting and bent over exercises. All exercises should have back in neutral, stable position, except those which specifically involve trunk movement.	Poor biomechanics can worsen existing problems. Any exercises that cause pain should be eliminated. Movements should be performed slowly. Minimize or eliminate unsupported forward flexion exercises in standing position. Avoid higher-risk exercises such as double leg raises, V-sits, or full sit-ups. Teach proper body mechanics, especially when lifting.

	Exercise Prescription	Exercise Precautions
Coronary artery disease	Goal: participate in multiple activities that maximize the carryover of training benefits to real-life activities. Frequency: 3–5 times/week. Duration: 30–60% peak HR. Intensity: 11–14 on RPE.	Cardiac symptoms should be disease stable or absent; medications limiting cardiac output use RPE to gauge intensity. Emphasize adequate warm-up and cool-down. May require physician oversight.
Osteoarthritis	Emphasize minimal, non–weight-bearing activities and interval activities. Modified stretching program. Low-resistance, low-repetition strength training. Warm-water exercise beneficial. Goal: maintain ROM on pain free days.	Participants with difficulty in joint mobility in hips or knees, movements down and up from floor may be contraindicated. Calisthenics should be prescribed with care.
Pregnancy	Stop exercising when fatigued and do not exercise to exhaustion. Non–weight-bearing exercises may be preferable. Use RPE to monitor intensity. Perform abdominals in alternative positions, such as standing, all fours, or side-lying position after first trimester. Be sure rectus abdominis is activated by performing spinal flexion in these positions.	Avoid exercise in supine position after first trimester. Avoid exercises where there is potential for loss of balance or abdominal stress. Avoid Valsalva maneuver. Ensure adequate hydration and nutrition.
Elderly	Recognize individual differences in fitness levels. Focus on safety; longer warm-up and cool-down. Emphasize moderate strength training and flexibility exercises. Emphasize exercises that relate to activities of daily living. Include exercises for balance.	Movements should be performed slowly. Consider minimal or non–weight-bearing activities if senior has musculoskeletal limitations. Important to know the medications and possible contraindications with exercise.

American College of Obstetricians and Gynecologists (ACOG, 1994) Recommendations for Exercise During Pregnancy and Postpartum

1. During pregnancy, women can continue to exercise and derive health benefits even from mild to moderate exer-

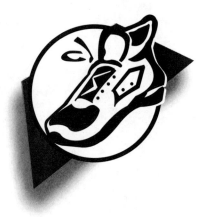

cise routines. Regular exercise (at least 3 times a week) is preferable to intermittent activity.

2. Women should avoid exercise in the supine position after the first trimester. Such a position is associated with decreased cardiac output in most pregnant women. Because the remaining cardiac output will be preferentially distributed away from splanchnic beds (including the uterus) during vigorous exercise, such regimens are best avoided during pregnancy. Prolonged periods of motionless standing should also be avoided.

3. Women should be aware of the decreased oxygen available for aerobic exercise during pregnancy. They should be encouraged to modify the intensity of their exercise according to maternal symptoms. Pregnant women should stop exercising when they are fatigued and not exercise to exhaustion. Under some circumstances, weight-bearing exercises may be continued throughout pregnancy at intensities similar to those before pregnancy. Non–weight-bearing exercises, such as cycling or swimming, will minimize the risk of injury and facilitate the continuation of exercise during pregnancy.

4. Morphologic changes in pregnancy should serve as a relative contraindication to types of exercise in which loss of balance could be detrimental to maternal or fetal well-being, especially in the third trimester. Furthermore, any type of exercise involving the potential for even mild abdominal trauma should be avoided.

5. Pregnancy requires an additional 300 kcal/day to maintain metabolic homeostasis. Thus, women who exercise during pregnancy should be particularly careful to ensure that their diets are adequate.

6. Women who exercise in the first trimester should augment heat dissipation by ensuring adequate hydration, wearing appropriate clothing, and exercising in an optimal environment.

7. Many of the physiologic and morphologic changes of pregnancy persist 4 to 6 weeks postpartum. Thus, pregnancy exercise routines should be resumed gradually based on a woman's physical capability.

Reasons to Discontinue Exercise and Seek Medical Advice During Pregnancy

1. Any signs of bloody discharge from the vagina.
2. Any gush of fluid from the vagina (premature rupture of membranes).
3. Sudden swelling of ankles, hands, or face.
4. Persistent, severe headaches and/or visual disturbance; unexplained spell of faintness or dizziness.

5. Swelling, pain, and redness in the calf of one leg (phlebitis).

6. Elevation of pulse rate or blood pressure that persists after exercise.

7. Excessive fatigue, palpitations, or chest pain.

8. Persistent contractions (more than 6–8/hour) that may suggest onset of premature labor.

9. Unexplained abdominal pain.

10. Insufficient weight gain (less than 1.0 kg/month during the last two trimesters).

Exercise Modifications

The following is a list of the major muscle groups, the action performed, and one example of an exercise with modifications for the special population indicated. The intent of this chart is to provide the candidate with a sample of the numerous possibilities for specific exercise modifications.

Muscle	Action	Special Populations/ Conditions	Exercise Modification
Hamstrings	Knee flexion	Aging, obesity, hypertension, pregnancy	Additional support. Light to no resistance. Should not lie on stomach or back during 2nd and 3rd trimester.
	Stretching	Low back pain	Supine with knees flexed and flat on the floor, bring one knee to chest, extend knee, provide gentle support on the back of thigh and hold stretch. No pain should be experienced.
Quadriceps	Knee extension	Aging, obesity, youth, low back pain, pregnancy, osteoarthritis	Postural considerations for low back pain. Light resistance. Caution with range-of-motion (ROM) (hyperextension) leg extensions. Hands on thighs for squats to minimize low back stress.

continued

ACSM HEALTH & FITNESS TRACK CERTIFICATIONS

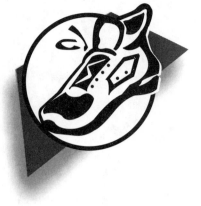

Muscle	Action	Special Populations/ Conditions	Exercise Modification
	Stretching	Same as above	Standing, support for balance, hold leg curl position, with knee pointing straight down to floor, hip and knee in alignment (neutral position). Caution with lordotic curve (hyperextension). Keep abdominals tight and do not hold breath.
Iliopsoas	Hip flexion	Low back pain, pregnancy, obesity, osteoarthritis, aging	Stretching is important to minimize the lordotic curve. Provide additional support for balance.
	Stretching		In modified forward lunge, support is on front leg, with weight over heel of front leg, up on ball of back foot; maintain a posterior pelvic tilt, contract abdominals and do not hold breath.
Gluteus maximus	Hip extension	Low back pain, pregnancy, obesity, osteoarthritis, aging	Support for balance. Caution with lordotic curve (hyperextension). Slow, controlled movement, limit ROM.
Hip abductors	Hip abduction	Low back pain, pregnancy, aging, obesity, osteoarthritis	Use side-lying position. Neutral spine. Avoid lateral flexion of trunk during movement. Limit ROM.
	Stretching	Low back pain, pregnancy, youth	Provide low back support. Limit ROM. Maintain shoulder and hip alignment. Do not hold breath. Seated position: one leg extended on floor, one leg bent with foot flat on floor; using opposite arm, gently pull tight toward midline of the body and hold stretch.

32

Muscle	Action	Special Populations/ Conditions	Exercise Modification
Hip adductors	Hip adduction	Low back pain, pregnancy, obesity, osteoarthritis, aging	Side-lying position. Neutral spine. Hips stacked. Top foot medial arch on floor in front of body, bottom leg lifts above midline of body with the head on upper arm and neck in neutral position.
Gastro-cnemius	Plantar flexion	Low back pain, obesity, aging, osteoarthritis	Avoid hyperextending knees. Maintain neutral posture, support for balance. Heel lifts (calf raises).
	Stretching	Same as above	Support for balance. Contract abdominals, do not hold breath. With forward lunge, caution with distance between front and back foot, weight on front foot. Use caution with knee alignment over heel. Provide a wide base of support with back heel maintaining contact with floor and hold stretch.
Anterior tibialis	Dorsiflexion	Low back pain, pregnancy, obesity	Avoid hyperextending knee (if standing). Support for balance. Maintain neutral position standing with knees slightly bent. Lift toes up toward body, heels maintain contact with floor.
Rectus abdominis	Spinal flexion	Low back pain, pregnancy, obesity	Precautions for hyper-flexion of cervical spine. Support for balance. Standing with knees bent, wide base of support, hands on thighs, pelvic tilt, contract abdominals, and do not hold breath. Spinal flexion exercises can also be given in the side-lying and all fours positions.

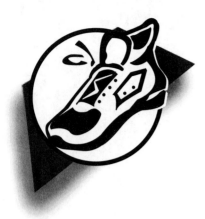

■ **REFERENCES**

ACSM. *ACSM's Guidelines for Exercise Testing and Prescription.* 6th ed. Baltimore: Lippincott Williams & Wilkins, 2000.

ACSM. *ACSM's Resource Manual for Guidelines for Exercise Testing and Prescription.* 3rd ed. Baltimore: Williams & Wilkins, 1998.

ACSM. *ACSM's Exercise Management for Persons with Chronic Diseases and Disabilities.* Champaign, IL: Human Kinetics, 1997.

Aerobics and Fitness Association of America. *Fitness: Theory & Practice.* 2nd ed. Sherman Oaks, CA: Aerobics and Fitness Association of America, 1995.

Anderson B. *Stretching.* Bolinas, CA: Shelter Publications, 1980.

Baechle TR, Groves BR. *Essentials of Strength Training and Conditioning.* Champaign, IL: Human Kinetics, 1994.

Cailliet R. *Understand Your Backache.* Philadelphia: FA Davis, 1987.

Cotton R, ed. *Aerobics Instructor Manual: The Resource for Fitness Professionals.* San Diego, CA: American Council on Exercise, 1993.

Fleck SJ, Kraemer WJ. *Designing Resistance Training Programs.* Champaign, IL: Human Kinetics, 1997.

Franks BD, Howley ET. *Fitness Leaders' Handbook.* Champaign, IL: Human Kinetics, 1989.

Kennedy C, Legel D. *Anatomy of an Exercise Class: An Exercise Educators' Handbook.* Champaign, IL: Sagamore Publishing, 1992.

Noble E. *Essential Exercises for the Childbearing Years.* 3rd ed. Boston: Houghton Mifflin, 1998.

Rimmer JH. *Fitness and Rehabilitation Programs for Special Populations.* Dubuque, IA: Wm. C. Brown & Benchmark, 1994.

Westcott W. *Strength Fitness.* 3rd ed. Dubuque, IA: Wm. C. Brown & Benchmark, 1991.

Yoke MM. *A Guide to Personal Fitness Training.* Sherman Oaks, CA: Aerobics and Fitness Association of America, 1997.

ACSM Health/Fitness Instructor SM Certification

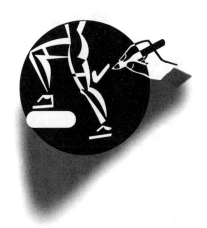

The ACSM Health/Fitness Instructor$_{SM}$ (H/FI) is a professional qualified to assess, design, and implement individual and group exercise and fitness programs for apparently healthy individuals and individuals with controlled disease. The H/FI is skilled in evaluating health behaviors and risk factors, conducting fitness assessments, writing appropriate exercise prescriptions, and motivating individuals to modify negative health habits and maintain positive lifestyle behaviors for health promotion. Successful completion of the ACSM Health/Fitness Instructor$_{SM}$ certification process includes demonstrating competency through a written examination and a multistation practical examination. Certification is granted to candidates who successfully complete both examinations.

MINIMUM REQUIREMENTS AND RECOMMENDED COMPETENCIES

Minimum Requirements

➤ A 2-year, 4-year, or Masters degree in a health-related field from a regionally accredited college/university (verification by transcript or copy of degree)

OR

➤ Current enrollment, as a junior or higher in a degree granting health-related field from a regionally accredited college/university

OR

➤ A minimum of 900 hours of practical experience in a fitness setting

AND

➤ Have current cardiopulmonary resuscitation (CPR) certification.

Recommended Competencies

1. Demonstrate competence in the KSAs required of the ACSM Health/Fitness Instructor$_{SM}$ and ACSM Exercise Leader® as listed in the 6th edition of *ACSM's Guidelines for Exercise Testing and Prescription.*

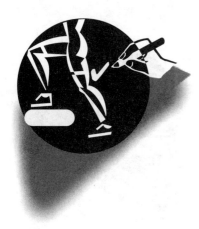

2. Have work-related experience within the health and fitness field.

3. Adequate knowledge of and skill in risk factor and health status identification, fitness appraisal, and exercise prescription.

4. Demonstrated ability to incorporate suitable and innovative activities that improve functional capacity.

5. Demonstrated ability to effectively educate and/or counsel individuals regarding lifestyle modification.

6. The ability to organize and administer health and fitness programs for a wide range of individuals with no known disease or with controlled disease.

7. Knowledge of exercise science including kinesiology, functional anatomy, exercise physiology, nutrition, program administration, psychology, and injury prevention.

WORKSHOP INFORMATION

A multiday workshop may be conducted in conjunction with the ACSM Health/Fitness Instructor$_{SM}$ certification examination. The purpose of the workshop is to provide a forum for acquiring new knowledge and updating techniques and skills. Workshops are not a prerequisite for certification, nor are they intended to provide the full experience and knowledge necessary for the successful completion of the examination. Workshops provide both a review of the Knowledge, Skills, and Abilities (KSAs) of the ACSM Health/Fitness Instructor$_{SM}$ and a forum for the acquisition of new knowledge and skills.

Participants should have prior experience and competence in monitoring heart rate (HR) and blood pressure (BP) both at rest and during exercise. BP training sessions are usually available from the local chapter of the American Heart Association if additional training is warranted. Experience in leading an exercise class, basic counseling skills, knowledge of functional anatomy, and knowledge of exercise physiology are also expected before attendance.

CERTIFICATION INFORMATION

Written Examination

The written examination contains approximately 100 multiple choice questions drawn from the KSAs in Appendix F in the 6th edition of *ACSM's Guidelines for Exercise Testing and Prescription*. KSAs outline minimal competencies necessary for certification. The table below lists the approximate number of questions from each of the areas represented by KSAs.

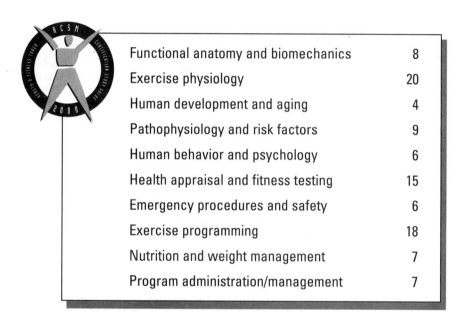

Functional anatomy and biomechanics	8
Exercise physiology	20
Human development and aging	4
Pathophysiology and risk factors	9
Human behavior and psychology	6
Health appraisal and fitness testing	15
Emergency procedures and safety	6
Exercise programming	18
Nutrition and weight management	7
Program administration/management	7

Sample Questions/Answers

The following sample questions are designed to help the candidate assess his or her knowledge base in preparation for the written portion of the ACSM Health/Fitness Instructor$_{SM}$ examination. The questions reflect the type of questions asked and the depth of knowledge expected. The answers follow the last question. Candidates are encouraged to review, in detail, those topics for which his or her answers were incorrect.

1. Which statement **best** reflects good technique for picking a barbell up from the floor?
   a. Lift with your back and upper body.
   b. Lift with your legs, keep your back straight, and keep the weight close to your body.
   c. Lift with your upper body and keep your back slightly rounded.
   d. Lift the weight quickly with your legs and back.

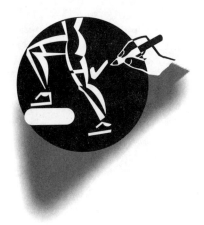

2. George is 50 years old, with a resting heart rate of 70 beats/min and a maximal heart rate of 178 beats/min. Using the Heart Rate Reserve (Karvonen) method for calculations, what is George's target heart rate at 75% of heart rate reserve as he exercises in your program?

  a. 136 beats/min
  b. 144 beats/min
  c. A 10-second pulse of 21
  d. A 10-second pulse of 25

3. Hypertension may be the result of which of the following?

  a. Heart disease
  b. Stress at work
  c. Genetic factors
  d. A combination of all of the above

4. The major muscle group used to flex the knee joint is the:

  a. quadriceps.
  b. hamstring.
  c. psoas major.
  d. biceps brachialis.
  e. none of the above.

5. Which item below indicates a high level of physical fitness for a 40-year-old man?

  a. Resting heart rate of 65 beats/min
  b. Sitting BP of 120/80 mm Hg
  c. Maximal aerobic power of 8 METs
  d. High-density lipoprotein of 45 mg/dL
  e. None of the above

6. Joan weighs 130 lbs. and has a measured maximal oxygen uptake of $42 \text{ mL} \cdot \text{kg}^{-1} \cdot \text{min}^{-1}$. What is her approximate energy cost to run a 6-mile distance in 54 minutes using 70% of her aerobic capacity?

  a. 8 kcal for each mile
  b. An average of 3.1 L of oxygen per mile
  c. 469 kcal
  d. 860 kcal

7. The amount of blood ejected from the heart with each beat is termed:

  a. stroke volume.
  b. ejection fraction.
  c. cardiac index.
  d. cardiac output.

8. A participant in your exercise class complained that during the night he experienced pain in the middle of his chest associated with a feeling of nausea and sweating. Although the pain has completely disappeared, he has reported his experience to you and intends to participate in your exercise session. What steps would you take with respect to the above information?

  a. Refer the participant to his physician.
  b. Carefully observe the participant during his exercise session that day.
  c. Consider the episode an epigastric problem and advise the participant to monitor it.
  d. Ask the participant to start exercising slowly and report any further discomfort.

9. An individual sprains his ankle while participating in your exercise class. You should have the individual:

    a. walk slowly until the pain in the injured ankle decreases.

    b. elevate his injured ankle and apply ice and compression.

    c. elevate his injured ankle and apply a warm compress.

    d. keep the injured ankle lower than the rest of the body and apply a warm compress.

10. Which of the following is **not** a beneficial physiological consequence of warm-up?

    a. Increased blood flow to muscle

    b. Increased muscle temperature

    c. Increase in oxygen consumption by the muscles

    d. Vasoconstriction of small blood vessels in the muscles

    e. All of the above

11. According to the ACSM, when providing a complete physical fitness assessment for a participant during a single testing session, what area of fitness should be assessed first?

    a. Aerobic capacity

    b. Body composition

    c. Flexibility

    d. Muscular fitness

12. Which of the following is **not** a reason to terminate a submaximal bicycle ergometer physical work capacity test?

    a. Malfunction of the metronome.

    b. Participant appears lightheaded and dizzy.

    c. Participant requests a stop, although there are no visible signs of discomfort.

    d. Systolic blood pressure is 226 mm Hg.

13. Multiple measurements at a single skinfold site should be taken until two or more measurements are within what range?

    a. 1 mm

    b. 2 mm

    c. 3 mm

    d. 4 mm

14. Which technique is least effective at improving your base of support during exercise?

    a. Widening your stance

    b. Choosing correct footwear

    c. Keeping weight close to your body whenever possible

    d. Elevating your center of gravity

15. A health/fitness instructor observes an individual performing an exercise incorrectly. Which of the following is the most effective teaching sequence?

    1. Reevaluate participant performance.

    2. Solicit feedback from participant.

    3. Demonstrate correct exercise execution.

    4. Have participant perform exercise.

    a. 1, 2, 3, 4

    b. 3, 4, 1, 2

    c. 2, 1, 4, 3

    d. 2, 3, 4, 1

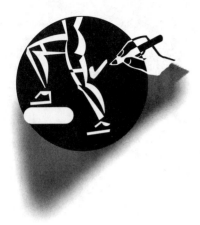

16. Of the following, the **least** effective motivational tool to encourage exercise compliance in an individual beginning an exercise program would be:

    a. providing alternative exercise modes.

    b. recording exercise progress.

    c. reviewing negative ramifications of physical inactivity.

    d. setting short-term goals.

17. A participant who is currently taking β-blockers will probably experience which of the following responses during submaximal exercise when compared with his or her response before beginning medication?

    a. Decrease in absolute VO_2

    b. Decrease in heart rate

    c. Decrease in tidal volume

    d. Increase in systolic BP

18. A participant at your facility has recently been diagnosed with type 2 diabetes. She has consulted with her physician and has received clearance to continue her exercise program. Which of the following documents is not necessary to include in the participant's file before resumption of her exercise program?

    a. Complete dietary analysis

    b. Orthopedic recommendation from appropriate health-care provider

    c. Physician recommendation regarding exercise intensity

    d. Recommended time and type of preexercise snacks

19. A 48-year-old female desires to start an exercise program in your facility. Following an initial questionnaire and interview you find that she has no personal history of heart disease, but her father died following a heart attack at the age of 60. In addition, she has a resting blood pressure of 145/85 mm Hg. Her total cholesterol is 220 mg/dL, with an HDL of 69 mg/dL. She is not obese. She currently walks for 30 minutes 4 times a week, but does not strength train. According to ACSM guidelines, this person would be classified as:

    a. apparently healthy.

    b. at increased risk.

    c. individual with known disease.

    d. none of the above.

20. Using the above example, which of the following is **true**?

    a. She should undergo a medical examination prior to starting a vigorous exercise program, and a physician should be available to supervise maximal exercise testing.

    b. She should undergo a medical examination prior to starting a vigorous exercise program, but it is not necessary for a physician to supervise maximal exercise testing.

    c. She does not need to undergo a medical examination prior to starting a vigorous exercise program. If she decides to have a maximal exercise test, a physician should be available to supervise.

    d. She does not need to undergo a medical examination prior to starting a vigorous exercise program. If she decides to have a maximal exercise test, it is not required for a physician to be available to supervise.

21. During stage 2 of a YMCA submaximal bicycle ergometer test, if the 2-minute heart rate is 114 bpm and the 3-minute heart rate is 126 bpm, what would be an appropriate response?

    a. Terminate the test because of the large increase in heart rate indicating fatigue.
    b. The workload should be increased to the stage 3 workload.
    c. The workload should stay the same for an additional minute because steady state has not been achieved.
    d. The workload should be decreased to the previous level until steady state is achieved.

22. To develop a strategic program for a fitness facility, a needs assessment is often conducted. Which of the following methods is **not** a part of this assessment?

    a. Target market surveys
    b. Focus groups
    c. Member and staff feedback
    d. Equipment and supply costs

23. Understanding budget development and forecasting is most relevant to a health/fitness instructor because:

    a. fitness instructors often become fitness directors.
    b. fitness instructors may own a house and have a family.
    c. fitness instructors often develop programs and services that require cost/benefit analysis.
    d. fitness instructors are often asked for feedback on the management of clubs.

24. From a marketing perspective which of the following statements is **true**?

    a. "Sell the sizzle, not the steak" or design a program that you like and create a program to sell it.
    b. Identify what the market needs and develop a program that will meet those needs with quality service.
    c. People want bells and whistles and are less concerned with the basics.
    d. Good-looking trainers in tight outfits always sell better than well-educated trainers in professional outfits.

25. Once a facility develops a strong customer base, it can rely on word of mouth for growth instead of additional marketing, true or false?

    a. True, because word of mouth is your best marketing and spending more money is a waste
    b. False, because you always want to find new markets and develop new programs that will need promotion within the community

Answers

1.	b	8.	a	15.	d	22.	d
2.	d	9.	b	16.	c	23.	c
3.	d	10.	d	17.	b	24.	b
4.	b	11.	b	18.	a	25.	b
5.	e	12.	d	19.	a		
6.	c	13.	b	20.	d		
7.	a	14.	d	21.	c		

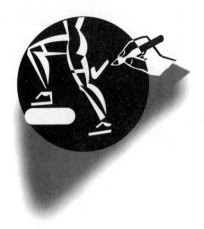

Practical Examination

The practical examination is composed of three separate test stations, each 20 minutes in length, for a total of 60 minutes. The practical examination is administered with consistency and uniformity throughout the certification sites. Time limitations are strictly enforced to ensure equity among candidates. Each of the practical stations is designed to be distinct and independent of all other practical examination stations. Candidates will be randomly assigned to start the practical examination at any one of the stations and will rotate through the remaining stations in numeric order. Candidates should arrive for testing 15 minutes before the start of their practical examination rotation.

Although many acceptable protocols exist in the field of fitness assessment, the protocols used in the practical examination are chosen as a representative sample of available, valid assessments. The selected protocols are included in this study guide. In this manner, both the candidate and the examiner know the expectations of the practical examination process. In some instances, the candidate may be asked to demonstrate only specific skills related to conducting the assessment rather than the entire protocol.

At each station, candidates will be evaluated on their knowledge and behavior in conducting assessments and skill/accuracy. Each item is individually weighted (i.e., assigned different points/percentages) in the calculation of a candidate's total score. Although some items are weighted higher than others, no one item is weighted so high as to allow a candidate to fail based solely on failure of that item. The candidate must fail a number of items to fail the examination. A failing score requires retesting of the entire practical examination. All examiners have current ACSM certification (H/FI or higher). An objective set of criteria and a standard script or scenario are used by each examiner. The examiner is not allowed to provide feedback or prompt further response. It is the responsibility of the candidate to respond concisely and appropriately to the scenario provided.

The practical examination will include evaluation in the following areas:

Body composition assessment

Exercise prescription development

Communication skills

Exercise demonstration and modification

Flexibility assessment

Muscular endurance assessment

Risk factor assessment

Preparing to conduct a physical work capacity (PWC) test

Conducting a PWC test

Before the examination, all certification candidates will have the opportunity to review the equipment that will be used. The site director or certification director at the testing site will provide the time schedule for review. Finalized practical examination schedules are usually prepared within 48 hours of the examination. If necessary, the candidate should check with the site director to confirm the practical examination schedule.

At the end of the practical examination, candidates are given the opportunity to meet with the certification director and complete an ACSM evaluation form anonymously. This is an opportunity for the candidate to provide the test site, the ACSM National Office, and the ACSM Committee on Certification and Education with information regarding the examination experience. The ACSM Health/Fitness Instructor$_{SM}$ certification is prepared by a number of leading professionals serving on the Health/Fitness Track Subcommittee, and these comments are considered carefully in the preparation and refinement of ACSM Health/Fitness Instructor$_{SM}$ certifications. Many of the changes that have been implemented in the ACSM Health/Fitness Instructor$_{SM}$ certification over the years have been in direct response to specific recommendations made by candidates.

Practical Examination Stations

Station 1. Body Composition, Flexibility, and Strength

A. Identify sites and demonstrate proper technique in estimating body composition using standard anthropometric protocols (including skinfold and circumference measurements).

Skinfold and Circumference Sites

■ Sources

ACSM. *ACSM's Guidelines for Exercise Testing and Prescription.* 6th ed. Baltimore: Lippincott Williams & Wilkins, 2000.
ACSM. *ACSM's Resource Manual for Guidelines for Exercise Testing and Prescription.* 3rd ed. Baltimore: Williams & Wilkins, 1998.

B. Demonstrate proper administration of the trunk flexion flexibility assessment.

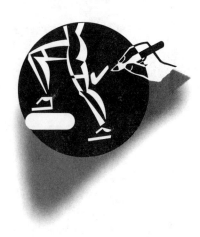

Trunk Flexion Sit-and-Reach Test Protocol

■ **SOURCES**

ACSM. *ACSM's Guidelines for Exercise Testing and Prescription.* 6th ed. Baltimore: Lippincott Williams & Wilkins, 2000.

ACSM. *ACSM's Resource Manual for Guidelines for Exercise Testing and Prescription.* 3rd ed. Baltimore: Williams & Wilkins, 1998.

Golding LA, Myers CR, Sinning WE. *The Y's Way to Fitness.* Champaign, IL: Human Kinetics, 1991.

> **C.** Demonstrate exercise instruction ability. Teach/demonstrate range of motion/flexibility exercises for specific muscle groups.

■ **SOURCES**

ACSM. *ACSM's Resource Manual for Guidelines for Exercise Testing and Prescription.* 3rd ed. Baltimore: Williams & Wilkins, 1998.

Baechle TR. *Essentials of Strength Training and Conditioning.* Champaign, IL: Human Kinetics, 1994.

American Council on Exercise. Group Fitness Instructor, Flexibility Training. 2/98.

> **D.** Demonstrate exercise instruction ability. Teach/demonstrate resistance training exercises for specific muscle group(s).

Push-up Endurance Test Protocol

■ **SOURCES**

ACSM. *ACSM's Resource Manual for Guidelines for Exercise Testing and Prescription.* 3rd ed. Baltimore: Williams & Wilkins, 1998.

Baechle TR. *Essentials of Strength Training and Conditioning.* Champaign, IL: Human Kinetics, 1994.

Station 2. Health/Fitness Consultation

> **A.** The candidate will be given health information and fitness testing results for review. They will then be expected to discuss these results with the client including the following information:

- Risk factors
- Risk stratification
- Identification of what values measured mean to the client including their present fitness categorization

- Goal fitness category discussed for each fitness value measured (body composition, cardiovascular, muscular strength and endurance, and flexibility)
- Exercise prescription based on frequency, intensity, time, type (include guidelines for cardiovascular, muscular strength and endurance, and flexibility)

Each candidate is given a worksheet. It is strongly recommended that you use the worksheet as a guide to keep on task and cover all required aspects.

■ SOURCES

ACSM. *ACSM's Guidelines for Exercise Testing and Prescription.* 6th ed. Baltimore: Lippincott Williams & Wilkins, 2000.
ACSM. *ACSM's Resource Manual for Guidelines for Exercise Testing and Prescription.* 3rd ed. Baltimore: Williams & Wilkins, 1998.
ACSM. *ACSM's Exercise Management for Persons with Chronic Diseases and Disabilities.* Champaign, IL: Human Kinetics, 1997.
Yoke MM. *A Guide to Personal Fitness Training.* Sherman Oaks, CA: Aerobics and Fitness Association of America, 1997.

Station 3. Preparation and Performance of Physical Work Capacity Test

> **A.** Discuss the necessary preparation for the testing site and equipment, including the following:

Emergency Procedures

■ SOURCES

ACSM. *ACSM's Guidelines for Exercise Testing and Prescription.* 6th ed. Baltimore: Lippincott Williams & Wilkins, 2000.
ACSM. *ACSM's Resource Manual for Guidelines for Exercise Testing and Prescription.* 3rd ed. Baltimore: Williams & Wilkins, 1998.

Testing Environment

■ SOURCES

ACSM. *ACSM's Guidelines for Exercise Testing and Prescription.* 6th ed. Baltimore: Lippincott Williams & Wilkins, 2000.
ACSM. *ACSM's Resource Manual for Guidelines for Exercise Testing and Prescription.* 3rd ed. Baltimore: Williams & Wilkins, 1998.

Preparation of Equipment

■ SOURCES

ACSM. *ACSM's Resource Manual for Guidelines for Exercise Testing and Prescription.* 3rd ed. Baltimore: Williams & Wilkins, 1998.

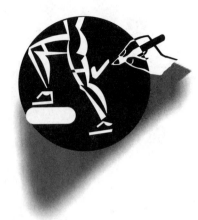

> **B.** Performing the physical work capacity (PWC) test, which includes the following:

Explain the Informed Consent of the PWC Test Including Explanation, Risks, Participant Responsibilities, and Benefits

■ **SOURCE**

ACSM. *ACSM's Guidelines for Exercise Testing and Prescription.* 6th ed. Baltimore: Lippincott Williams & Wilkins, 2000.

Explain the Rating of Perceived Exertion (RPE) Scale

■ **SOURCE**

ACSM. *ACSM's Guidelines for Exercise Testing and Prescription.* 6th ed. Baltimore: Lippincott Williams & Wilkins, 2000.

> **C.** Preparing the participant for testing on a bicycle ergometer, including the following:

Equipment Adjustments and Participant Position

■ **SOURCE**

Howley ET, Franks BD. Health Fitness Instructor Handbook. 2nd ed. Champaign, IL: Human Kinetics, 1997.

Measurement of Preexercise Heart Rate

■ **SOURCES**

ACSM. *ACSM's Resource Manual for Guidelines for Exercise Testing and Prescription.* 3rd ed. Baltimore: Williams & Wilkins, 1998.
Heyward VH. *Advanced Fitness Assessment & Exercise Prescription.* 2nd ed. Champaign, IL: Human Kinetics, 1991.

Measurement of Preexercise Blood Pressure

■ **SOURCES**

ACSM. *ACSM's Guidelines for Exercise Testing and Prescription.* 6th ed. Baltimore: Lippincott Williams & Wilkins, 2000.
ACSM. *ACSM's Resource Manual for Guidelines for Exercise Testing and Prescription.* 3rd ed. Baltimore: Williams & Wilkins, 1998.
American Heart Association. Recommendations for human blood pressure determination by sphygmomanometer. Dallas: National Center, 1987.

> **D.** Administer selected standardized bicycle ergometer submaximal PWC test developed for the Health/Fitness Instructor$_{SM}$ practical examination.

■ SOURCES

ACSM. *ACSM's Guidelines for Exercise Testing and Prescription.* 6th ed. Baltimore: Lippincott Williams & Wilkins, 2000.

Golding LA, Myer CR, Sinning WE. *The Y's Way to Fitness.* Champaign, IL: Human Kinetics, 1991.

The PWC protocol used in the Health/Fitness Instructor~SM~ practical examination is provided to the candidate at this station. The protocol will be a continuous, multistage, submaximal bicycle ergometer test with 3-minute stages. The termination heart rate (70% of heart rate reserve) will be provided to the candidate. The candidate will be asked to proceed with the PWC following the provided protocol to evaluate the following competencies:

1. Ability to demonstrate the proper transition to increasing work rates at appropriate times.
2. Ability to measure heart rate, blood pressure, and RPE during selected stages of the exercise test.
3. Ability to terminate the test when the individual reaches a steady state at 85% of age-predicted heart rate maximum (70% of heart rate reserve) or when signs or symptoms of distress occur (i.e., nausea, dizziness, unusual rise or fall in blood pressure).

Suggested PWC Practice Protocols

■ SOURCES

ACSM. Submaximal cycle ergometer protocols.
The Y's Way to Fitness: Physical Work Capacity Test. H/FI Study Guide.

ACSM Statement Regarding Health/Fitness Instructor~SM~ Protocol Selection

The protocols listed under the examination subject areas represent standardized protocols available in the field. They may be found in the resources listed for each protocol detailed in the study guide and/or in the reference section at the end of this study guide. At each station, where appropriate, the examiner will provide the candidate with a testing protocol from the previous listing. Although the protocol is available, the candidate should be completely familiar with each protocol before examination day. The testing period does not allow sufficient time for the candidate to review or study the protocol. Experience has shown that well-prepared candidates are familiar with the specific procedures. The ACSM is well aware that multiple protocols exist for most assessments with varying degrees of acceptance and popularity. Attention was paid to choosing protocols that are as well documented and as widely accepted as possible. ACSM is not endors-

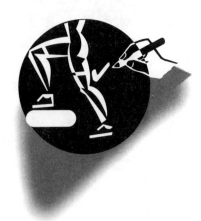

ing these protocols over others in the field. They were chosen simply to provide a degree of standardization and fairness to the examination process.

CERTIFICATION CONTENT MATERIAL

Standardized Description of Skinfold Measurements

Identification of Sites

Abdominal: a vertical fold taken at a distance 2 cm to the right side of the umbilicus.

Biceps: a vertical fold taken on the anterior aspect of the arm over the belly of the biceps muscle 1 cm above the level used to mark the triceps.

Calf (medial): a vertical fold at a level of the maximum circumference of the calf on the midline of its medial border.

Chest/pectoral: a diagonal fold taken half the distance between the anterior axillary line and the nipple (men) and one-third the distance between the anterior axillary line and the nipple (women).

Midaxillary: a vertical fold taken on the midaxillary line at the level of the xiphoid process of the sternum (an alternate method is a horizontal fold taken at the level of the xiphoid/sternal border in the midaxillary line).

Subscapular: a diagonal fold taken at a 45° angle 1 to 2 cm below the inferior angle of the scapula.

Suprailium: an oblique fold in line with the natural angle of the iliac crest taken in the anterior axillary line immediately superior to the iliac crest.

Thigh: a vertical fold on the anterior midline of the thigh, midway between the proximal border of the patella and the inguinal crease (hip).

Triceps: a vertical fold on the posterior midline of the upper right arm, halfway between the acromion and olecranon processes, with the arm held freely to the side of the body.

Procedures

1. Measurements should be taken on the right side of the body.
2. The caliper should be placed 1 cm away from the thumb and finger, perpendicular to the skinfold, and halfway between the crest and base of the fold.

3. Pinch should be maintained while reading the caliper; 1 to 2 seconds (and not longer) should elapse before reading the caliper.

4. Duplicate measures should be taken at each site.

5. If measurements do not fall within 1 to 2 mm of each other, they should be retaken.

6. The measurer should rotate through measurement sites or allow time for skin to regain normal texture and thickness.

7. The measurement is recorded when 2 consecutive measurements are within 1 to 2 mm of each other. Record the average between the two accepted values.

■ SOURCES

ACSM. *ACSM's Guidelines for Exercise Testing and Prescription.* 6th ed. Baltimore: Lippincott Williams & Wilkins, 2000.

ACSM. *ACSM's Resource Manual for Guidelines for Exercise Testing and Prescription.* 3rd ed. Baltimore: Williams & Wilkins, 1998.

Standardized Description of Circumference Measurements

Identification of Sites

Abdomen: With the subject relaxed, a horizontal measure taken at the level of the umbilicus.

Arm: With the arm to the side of the body, a horizontal measure taken midway between the acromion and olecranon processes.

Calf: With the subject standing erect, a horizontal measure taken at a level of the maximum circumference between the knee and the ankle.

Forearm: With the subject standing erect, with the arms hanging downward but slightly away from the trunk and the palms facing forward, the measure is taken perpendicular to the long axis of the forearm at the level of its maximum circumference.

Hips/buttocks: With the subject standing erect, a horizontal measure taken at the maximum circumference of the hips/buttocks region, whichever is larger (above the gluteal fold). The individual should be wearing a thin swimsuit or briefs. The measurer should squat at the side of the individual so that maximum extension of the buttocks can be seen.

Hips/thighs: With the legs slightly apart, a horizontal measure taken at the maximum circumference of the hips/thigh of the right leg, just below the gluteal fold.

Waist: With the abdomen relaxed, a horizontal measure taken at the level of the narrowest part of the torso (above the umbilicus and below the xiphoid process).

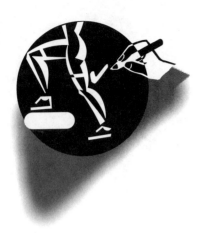

Procedures

1. Measurements should be taken on the right side of the body using a tension-regulated tape measure.
2. The tape measure should be placed perpendicular to the long axis of the body part.
3. The tape measure should be pulled to the proper tension without pinching the skin.
4. Duplicate measures should be taken at each site.
5. If measurements do not fall within 7 mm or (0.25 inches) of each other, they should be retaken.
6. The measurement is recorded when 2 consecutive measurements are taken that fall within 7 mm or 0.25 inches. Record the average between the 2 accepted values.

■ SOURCES

ACSM. *ACSM's Guidelines for Exercise Testing and Prescription.* 6th ed. Baltimore: Lippincott Williams & Wilkins, 2000.

ACSM. *ACSM's Resource Manual for Guidelines for Exercise Testing and Prescription.* 3rd ed. Baltimore: Williams & Wilkins, 1998.

Trunk Flexion—Sit-and-Reach Test Protocol

Purpose

To measure trunk forward flexion and determine hip, low back, and hamstring range of motion.

Equipment

1. A standard sit-and-reach box or yardstick.
2. Tape to keep yardstick on the floor.
3. Exercise mat.

Procedures

1. Participant should perform a short warm-up before this test. It is also recommended that the participant refrain from fast, jerky movements that may increase the possibility of injury. Shoes should be removed.
2. Place the yardstick on the floor, and tape across it at right angles to the 15-inch mark. The participant should sit with the yardstick between the legs and with the legs extended. Heels of the feet should touch near the edge of the taped line and be about 10 to 12 inches apart. If a standard sit-and-reach box is available, heels should be placed against the edge of the box.
3. The participant should slowly reach forward with both hands as far as possible on the yardstick, holding this

position momentarily. The tester should be sure that the participant keeps the hands parallel and does not stretch or lead with one hand. Fingertips can be overlapped and should be in contact with the yardstick or measuring portion of the sit-and-reach box.

4. The score is the most distant point (in inches) reached on the yardstick with the fingertips. The best of three trials should be recorded. To assist with the best attempt, the tester should suggest that the participant exhale and drop the head between the arms when reaching. Testers should ensure that the knees of the participant are kept straight. The participant's knees should not be pressed down by the tester.

Caution: The participant should not perform the Valsalva maneuver and should breathe easily during the exercise.

■ **SOURCES**

ACSM. *ACSM's Guidelines for Exercise Testing and Prescription.* 6th ed. Baltimore: Lippincott Williams & Wilkins, 2000.

ACSM. *ACSM's Resource Manual for Guidelines for Exercise Testing and Prescription.* 3rd ed. Baltimore: Williams & Wilkins, 1998.

Golding LA, Myers CR, Sinning WE. *The Y's Way to Fitness.* Champaign, IL: Human Kinetics, 1991.

Coronary Artery Disease Risk Factors

For the coronary artery disease risk factors, read the chart on pages 14 and 15 of this study guide.

■ **SOURCE**

ACSM. *ACSM's Guidelines for Exercise Testing and Prescription.* 6th ed. Baltimore: Lippincott Williams & Wilkins, 2000.

Initial Risk Stratification

Individuals with the above risk factors face an increased risk of a cardiac crisis while exercising. Therefore, it is critical to determine risk and further classify in order to help the fitness instructor guide the participant to the best course of action before beginning an exercise program. The following risk stratification classifications are recommended for potential exercisers:

1. Apparently healthy: Individuals who are asymptomatic and apparently healthy with no more than one coronary risk factor (see table above).

2. Increased risk: Individuals who have signs or symptoms suggestive of possible cardiopulmonary or metabolic dis-

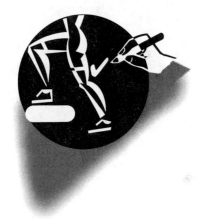

ease and/or two or more coronary risk factors (see table above).

3. Known disease: Individuals with known cardiac, pulmonary, metabolic disease.

ACSM Recommendations for Medical Examination and Exercise Testing Prior to Participation and Physician Supervision of Exercise Tests

Medical examination and clinical exercise test recommended prior to participation:

| | Apparently Healthy | | Increased Risk* | | |
	Younger	Older	No Symptoms	Symptoms	Known Disease**
Moderate Exercise[1]	No	No	No	Yes	Yes
Vigorous Exercise[2]	No	Yes	Yes	Yes	Yes

Physician supervision recommended during exercise test:

| | Apparently Healthy | | Increased Risk* | | |
	Younger	Older	No Symptoms	Symptoms	Known Disease**
Submaximal testing	No	No	No	Yes	Yes
Maximal testing	No	Yes	Yes	Yes	Yes

*Persons with two or more risk factors.
**Persons with known cardiac, pulmonary, or metabolic disease.
[1]Moderate exercise is defined by an intensity of 40% to 60% of $\dot{V}O_{2max}$ (50% to 70% of maximum heart rate).
[2]Vigorous exercise is defined by an intensity > 60% $\dot{V}O_{2max}$ (> 70% of maximum heart rate).
Source: *ACSM's Guidelines for Exercise Testing and Prescription.* 6th ed. Baltimore: Lippincott Williams & Wilkins, 2000.

Medications

Many individuals who exercise also take medications for a variety of medical and physical conditions. Certain medications affect the heart rate and/or blood pressure at rest and during exercise (reduction in resting and exercise heart rate will interfere with heart rate as a measure of intensity). Some medications may have an effect on exercise capacity (reduction in exercise capacity may require a change in the exercise prescription) and in some cases may cause a negative effect (contraindication) during exercise (one should not exercise while using these medications). Because of these possible effects, it is critical that the health/fitness instructor know the medications used by the participant and understands the effects of those medications during exercise. Listed below are some of the classifications of medications and their effect on heart rate, blood pressure, and exercise capacity.

Medications	Heart Rate	Blood Pressure	Exercise Capacity
β-Blockers	Decrease (resting and exercise)	Decrease (resting and exercise)	Increase with angina No change without angina
Nitrates	Increase resting Increase or no change with exercise	Decrease resting Decrease or no change with exercise	Increase with angina No change without angina
Calcium channel blockers	Increase or no change (resting and exercise)	Decrease (resting and exercise)	Increase with angina No change without angina
Diuretics	No change	Decrease or no change (resting and exercise)	No change, except with congestive heart failure (CHF)
ACE inhibitors	No change	Decrease (resting and exercise)	No change, except increase or no change with CHF
Vasodilators	Increase or no change	Decrease (resting and exercise)	No change, except increase or no change with CHF
Bronchodilators	No change	No change	Increase with people limited by bronchospasm
Antidepressants	Increase or no change (resting and exercise)	Decrease or no change	Variable
Prozac	Increase or no change	Increase or no change	Variable. May cause fatigue and poor balance
Lithium	No change	No change	May result in T-wave changes and arrhythmias

Blood Pressure Measurement

Blood pressure (BP) is a measure of the force or pressure exerted by the blood on the arteries. The highest measure, called the systolic BP, is the pressure on the arteries when the heart contracts. The lowest measure, called diastolic BP, occurs when the heart relaxes and is refilling with blood.

Positioning

1. The participant should be seated.
2. The arm should be fully supported at the level of the heart.
3. The elbow should be flexed at 45°.
4. The hand should be relaxed.

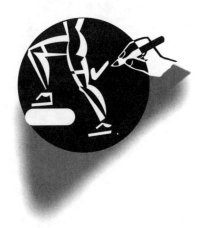

Application of Cuff and Stethoscope

1. The proper cuff size should be selected. The bladder should cover approximately two-thirds of the upper arm.
2. The cuff should be snug, with the center of the bladder over the brachial artery.
3. The lower edge of the cuff should be 2 to 3 cm above the antecubital space.
4. The stethoscope eartips should be adjusted so they face forward.
5. The stethoscope bell should be placed over the brachial artery. The artery can be found near (above or below) the antecubital fossa (crease created by the elbow joint on the inside of the arm). The brachial artery is located on the medial aspect of the arm.

Note: Use of undersized cuffs is one of the most common errors made during BP measurement. An undersized cuff distorts BP an average of 8.5 mm Hg for systolic and 4.6 mm Hg for diastolic readings (although errors can be much greater). Remember, the bladder should cover approximately two-thirds of the upper arm.

Preparation of Participants

1. The participant should receive an explanation about the measurement and be warned about mild discomfort that may be experienced.
2. The participant should sit and rest for 5 to 10 minutes before measurement.
3. The participant should not cross his or her legs or talk during the measurement.
4. The participant should wear loose clothing, especially around the upper arm; short sleeves are preferred.

Resting BP

1. After the appropriate preparation, the participant should be seated for at least 5 minutes with the elbow slightly flexed.
2. The cuff should be wrapped firmly around the upper arm at heart level and aligned with the brachial artery.
3. The stethoscope bell should be placed over the brachial artery.
4. The cuff pressure should be quickly inflated to 200 mm Hg or 20 to 30 mm Hg above the estimated systolic BP.
5. The pressure should be released slowly, at a rate equal to 2 to 3 mm Hg/sec, noting first Korotkoff sound (appearance of a clear pulse sound).

6. While continuing to release the pressure, it should be noted when sound becomes muffled (fourth Korotkoff phase diastolic BP) or when the sound disappears (fifth Korotkoff phase diastolic BP).

Potential Sources of Error in BP Measurement

1. Inaccurate sphygmomanometer.
2. Improper cuff size.
3. Auditory acuity of technician.
4. Rate of inflation or deflation of cuff pressure.
5. Experience of technician.
6. Reaction time of technician.
7. Improper stethoscope placement or pressure.
8. Background noise.
9. Patient holding treadmill handrails.
10. Certain physiological abnormalities (e.g., damaged brachial artery, subclavian steal syndrome, a-v fistula).

Sample Informed Consent for a Health-Related Exercise Test

1. *Explanation of the exercise test.*
   You will perform an exercise test on a cycle ergometer or a motor-driven treadmill. The exercise intensity will begin at a level you can easily maintain and will be advanced in stages depending on your fitness level. We may stop the test at any time because of signs of fatigue or you may stop when you wish because of personal feelings of fatigue or discomfort

2. *Risks and discomforts.*
   There exists the possibility of certain changes occurring during the test. These include abnormal blood pressure, fainting, disorder of heart beat, and in rare instances heart attack, stroke, or death. Every effort will be made to minimize these risks by evaluation of preliminary information relating to your health and fitness and by observations during the test. Emergency equipment and trained personnel are available to deal with unusual situations that may arise.

3. *Responsibilities of the participant.*
   Information you possess about your health status or previous experiences of unusual feelings with physical effort may affect the safety and value of your exercise test. Your prompt reporting of feelings with effort during the exercise test itself are also of great importance. You are responsible for fully disclosing such information when requested by the testing staff.

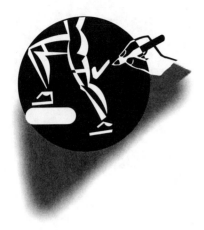

4. *Benefits to be expected.*
The results obtained from the exercise test may assist in diagnosing your illness or in evaluating what type of physical activities you might perform with low risk of harm.

5. *Inquiries.*
Any questions about the procedures used in the exercise test or in the estimation of functional capacity are encouraged. If you have any doubts or questions, please ask us for further explanations.

6. *Freedom of consent.*
Your permission to perform this exercise test is voluntary. You are free to deny consent or stop the test at any point, if you so desire.

I have read this form and I understand the test procedures that I will perform. I consent to participate in the test.

Participant's Signature/Date _____

Witness's Signature/Date _____

Tester's Signature/Date _____

■ SOURCES

ACSM. *ACSM's Guidelines for Exercise Testing and Prescription.* 6th ed. Baltimore: Lippincott Williams & Wilkins, 2000.

Standardized Guidelines for Submaximal Cardiovascular Evaluation

1. The submaximal PWC test is performed on a bicycle ergometer. The exercise test should begin with a 2- to 3-minute warm-up stage to orient the participant with the bicycle ergometer and prepare the participant for the exercise intensity that is initiated in the first stage of the exercise test.

2. The specific protocol is provided to the candidate and will consist of 3-minute stages with appropriate increments in work rate.

3. The participant should be positioned properly on the bicycle ergometer (i.e., upright posture, slight bend (5° to 10°) in the knee during extension, hands in proper position on handlebars).

4. Heart rate should be monitored at least 2 times during each stage using techniques recommended by Heyward (1991) and *ACSM's Resource Manual for Guidelines for Exercise Testing and Prescription,* 3rd ed. (1998). Measurements should be taken during the latter portions

of the second and third minutes of each stage. If heart rate is greater than 110 beats/min, steady-state heart rate (i.e., 2 heart rates within 6 beats/min) should be reached before workloads are increased.

5. Blood pressure should be monitored during the latter portions of each stage using techniques described by the American Heart Association (1987) and *ACSM's Resource Manual for Guidelines for Exercise Testing and Prescription,* 3rd ed. (1998).

6. RPE should be monitored at the latter portions of each stage using either the 6–20 Category Scale or the 0–10 Category-Ratio Scale.

7. Participant appearance and symptoms should be monitored regularly.

8. The exercise test should be terminated when the participant reaches 85% of age-predicted maximal heart rate (70% of heart rate reserve), fails to conform to the exercise test protocol, or experiences signs of discomfort or an emergency situation.

9. An appropriate cool-down/recovery period should be initiated consisting of either:

   A. An active recovery stage with the workload adjusted to a work rate equivalent to the first stage of the exercise test protocol or less; or

   B. A passive cool-down/recovery if the participant experiences signs of discomfort or an emergency situation in which the participant is unable to perform an active cool-down/recovery workload.

10. All observations (heart rate, BP, RPE, participant signs and symptoms) should be continued for at least 4 minutes of recovery unless abnormal responses occur that would require a longer post-test observation.

■ SOURCES

ACSM. *ACSM's Guidelines for Exercise Testing and Prescription.* 6th ed. Baltimore: Lippincott Williams & Wilkins, 2000.

Physical Work Capacity Test (1)

Very Active? (20 minutes aerobic exercise 3 days/week)	No	Yes
<169 lb	Protocol A	Protocol A
161–199 lb	Protocol A	Protocol B
>200 lb	Protocol B	Protocol C

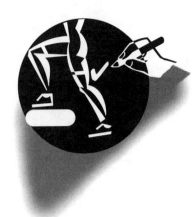

Work Loads (kgm/min) for Submaximal Test

Protocol	Stage I	Stage II	Stage III	Stage IV
A	150	300	450	600
B	150	300	600	900
C	300	600	900	1200

Note: 3-minute stages will be used in the practical examination.

See Standardized Guidelines for Administering the PWC test in this study guide.

Physical Work Capacity Test (2)

Stage I	150 kgm/min (0.5 kg)			
Warm-up	*HR < 80*	*HR 80–89*	*HR 90–100*	*HR > 100*
Stage II	750 kgm/min (2.5 kg)	600 kgm/min (2.0 kg)	450 kgm/min (1.5 kg)	300 kgm/min (1.0 kg)
Stage III	900 kgm/min (3.0 kg)	750 kgm/min (2.5 kg)	600 kgm/min (2.0 kg)	450 kgm/min (1.5 kg)
Stage IV	1050 kgm/min (3.5 kg)	900 kgm/min (3.0 kg)	750 kgm/min (2.5 kg)	600 kgm/min (2.0 kg)

Ratings of Perceived Exertion (RPE) Scales

Category Scale		Category-Ratio Scale	
6	Very, very light	0	Nothing at all
7		0.5	Very, very weak
8		1	Very Weak
9	Very light	2	Weak
10		3	Moderate
11	Fairly light	4	Somewhat strong
12		5	Strong
13	Somewhat hard	6	
14		7	Very strong
15	Hard	8	
16		9	
17	Very hard	10	Very, very strong
18		>10	Maximal
19	Very, very hard		
20			

■ REFERENCES

ACSM. *ACSM's Guidelines for Exercise Testing and Prescription.* 6th ed. Baltimore: Lippincott Williams & Wilkins, 2000.

ACSM. *ACSM's Resource Manual for Guidelines for Exercise Testing and Prescription.* 3rd ed.. Baltimore: Williams & Wilkins, 1998.

ACSM. *Exercise Management for Persons with Chronic Diseases and Disabilities.* Champaign, IL: Human Kinetics, 1997.

Alter S. *Science of Flexibility.* Champaign, IL: Human Kinetics, 1994.

American Heart Association. Recommendations for human blood pressure determination by sphygmomanometers. Dallas: National Center, 1987.

Baechle TR. *Essentials of Strength Training and Conditioning.* Champaign, IL: Human Kinetics, 1994.

Gavin RS, Gavin BE. *Psychology for Health Fitness Professionals.* Champaign, IL: Human Kinetics, 1995.

Golding LA, Meyers CR, Sinning WE. *The Y's Way to Fitness.* Champaign, IL: Human Kinetics, 1991.

Grantham WC, Patton RW, York TD, et al. *Health Fitness Management.* Champaign, IL: Human Kinetics, 1998.

Hamill J, Knutzen KM. *Biomechanical Basis of Human Movement.* Baltimore: Williams & Wilkins, 1995.

Howley ET, Franks BD. *Health/Fitness Instructor Handbook.* Champaign, IL: Human Kinetics, 1997.

Kendall FP, McCreary EK, Provance PG. *Muscles: Testing and Function.* 4th ed. Baltimore: Williams & Wilkins, 1993.

Lohman T, Roche AF, Martorell R, eds. *Anthropometric Standardization Reference Manual.* Abridged ed. Champaign, IL: Human Kinetics, 1991.

Nieman DC. *The Sports Medicine Fitness Course.* Palo Alto, CA: Bull Publishing, 1990.

Skinner JS. *Exercise Testing and Exercise Prescription for Special Cases.* 2nd ed. Baltimore: Williams & Wilkins, 1997.

Spence AP, Mason EB. *Anatomy and Physiology.* Redwood City, CA: Benjamin-Cummings, 1979.

Zigon ST. *How to Use the ACSM Metabolic Equations.* Canton, OH: Professional Reports, 1990.

ACSM Health/Fitness Director® Certification

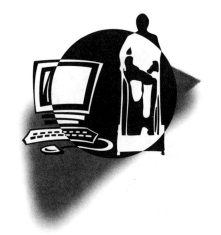

The ACSM Health/Fitness Director® certification provides professionals with recognition of their practical experience and demonstrated competence as an administrative leader of a health & fitness programs in the corporate, clinical, commercial, or community setting. These programs serve an apparently healthy population participating in health promotion and fitness-related activities. The professional responsibilities of an ACSM Health/Fitness Director® encompass an advanced knowledge of applied program administration, facility management, staff training and supervision, applied exercise physiology, and health-related issues.

MINIMUM REQUIREMENTS AND RECOMMENDED COMPETENCIES

Minimum Requirements

➤ A 2-year, 4-year, or Masters degree in a health-related field from a regionally accredited college/university (verification by transcript or copy of the degree); plus a minimum of 2 years (full-time) or 4000 hours of experience as a fitness manager or director

OR

➤ Current ACSM Health/Fitness Instructor$_{SM}$ certification plus 2 years (full-time) or 4000 hours of experience as a fitness manager or director

AND

➤ Have current cardiopulmonary resuscitation (CPR) certification.

Recommended Competencies

1. Demonstrate competence in the KSAs required of the ACSM Health/Fitness Director®, ACSM Health/Fitness Instructor$_{SM}$, and ACSM Exercise Leader® as listed in the 6th edition of *ACSM's Guidelines for Exercise Testing and Prescription*.
2. Demonstrate the practical skills in basic business organization and finance.

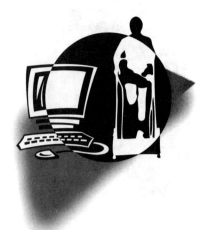

3. Demonstrate the ability to organize and administer health and fitness programs for a wide range of persons with no known disease or with controlled disease.

4. Possess knowledge and practical experience in the supervision and administration of health and fitness programs in a variety of settings. In addition, possess a knowledge of exercise science including kinesiology, functional anatomy, exercise physiology, nutrition, risk factor identification, fitness appraisal, lifestyle modification techniques, exercise prescription, and injury prevention.

WORKSHOP INFORMATION

Currently there is no ACSM workshop for this level of certification.

CERTIFICATION INFORMATION

The ACSM Health/Fitness Director® certification is granted to candidates successfully completing both the written and practical examinations.

Testing Information

Candidates should arrive a day in advance of the written or practical examination and be available for the entire scheduled testing period. Candidates must communicate directly with the site to obtain the testing schedule. Candidates must plan travel and accommodations accordingly.

Written Examination

The written examination contains approximately 100 multiple choice questions drawn from the KSAs in the 6th edition of *ACSM's Guidelines for Exercise Testing and Prescription*. KSAs outline the minimal competencies necessary for certification. The table below lists the approximate number of questions from each of the areas represented by KSAs. Candidates have 3 hours to complete the written exam.

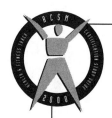

Functional anatomy and biomechanics	6
Exercise physiology	10
Human development and aging	5
Pathophysiology and risk factors	9
Human behavior and psychology	7
Health appraisal and fitness testing	8
Emergency procedures and safety	8
Exercise programming	10
Nutrition and weight management	7
Program administration/management	20
Health promotion	10

Sample Questions/Answers

The following sample questions are designed to assist the candidate in preparation for the written examination. The questions reflect both the type of questions asked and the depth of knowledge expected. The answers follow the last question. Candidates are encouraged to review, in detail, those topics for which his or her answers were incorrect.

1. The exercise area of a commercial fitness facility should take up what approximate percentage of the total square footage?
   a. 10 to 15%
   b. 30 to 45%
   c. 50 to 65%
   d. 70 to 85%

2. The coronary risk factors for which the most data exist to document an association with coronary disease are:
   a. obesity, hypercholesterolemia, and lack of exercise.
   b. smoking, hypertension, and hypercholesterolemia.
   c. stress, hypercholesterolemia, and hypertension.
   d. smoking, hypercholesterolemia, and lack of exercise.
   e. hypertension, hypercholesterolemia, and obesity.

3. Which of the following mechanical factors minimize the load placed on the lumbar spine when lifting a heavy weight?
   a. Flexing the knees
   b. Holding the object away from the body
   c. Inclining the trunk forward
   d. Looking down at the lifted weight

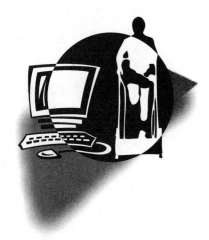

4. Which of the following is **false** regarding marketing and/or public relations?

   a. Marketing determines or creates the wants of people.
   b. Good marketing satisfies the wants and needs of people.
   c. Public relations builds a referral network.
   d. Public relations is frequently an expense item in the budget.

5. Which of the following is most true regarding profit assets and loss liabilities in various business enterprises?

   a. Co-owners in a partnership are personally protected by the business entity.
   b. A sole proprietorship spreads profits and liabilities to stockholders.
   c. Shareholders in an S-corporation are personally protected by the corporate entity.
   d. Personal retirement assets of a principal are subject to bankruptcy claims.

6. Which of the following is **most** true?

   a. Zero-based budgeting requires a short time for budget planning.
   b. Systems-approach budgeting allows for increased end-of-year spending.
   c. Incremental budgeting adjusts to the company's needs.
   d. Systems approach budgeting requires only a short time for budget planning.
   e. Zero-based budgeting adjusts to the company's needs.

7. Which method allows the ACSM Health/Fitness Director® to rapidly monitor participant facility use and screen eligible facility users?

   a. Computerized exercise log system
   b. Control desk area turnstile
   c. Sign-in sheet system
   d. Magnetic membership card reader system

8. In an advertising campaign to promote an employee fitness program, which method would ensure that the information would reach the greatest numbers?

   a. Memo
   b. Posted signs
   c. Group meetings
   d. Check stuffer

9. Which of the following data collection procedures would be incorporated into a program-efficiency evaluation of a fitness center?

   a. Check preprogram and postprogram changes in participants.
   b. Cost of program A compared with program B.
   c. Program effects on absenteeism.
   d. Check demographic description of participants.

10. The **most** reliable indicator of coronary artery disease is:

    a. substernal chest pain on exertion.
    b. total cholesterol to the high-density lipoprotein ratio of 5.5.
    c. negative graded exercise test.
    d. blood pressure readings of 210/100 mm Hg during exercise testing.

Answers

1. b	4. d	7. d	10. a
2. b	5. c	8. d	
3. a	6. e	9. b	

Practical Examination

The practical examination is designed to assess the ACSM Health/ Fitness Director® candidate in a context that attempts to simulate work-related situations in the areas of (1) business planning, (2) situational management, and (3) staff training. The examinations are not necessarily conducted in the aforementioned order for each candidate. The total examination time for each candidate on all 3 components is approximately 2 hours, distributed across 1 to 2 testing days, depending on the number of candidates and examiners involved. Stations are set up and scheduled to test candidates in an organized and efficient manner. Schedules are made available to all candidates and posted in appropriate testing areas. Casual business attire is appropriate and expected for this testing session.

Practical Examination Process

The examiners are certified ACSM Health/Fitness Director® or ACSM Program Director$_{SM}$. During the practical examination, a series of scenarios are presented to assess the candidate's ability to respond to work-related situations encountered by the typical ACSM Health/Fitness Director®. Candidates will have time to read and prepare a response for each scenario. Candidates are encouraged to bring a notepad and calculator to assist them in their response preparation. Following their response, the examiner will use a checklist to evaluate and record the candidates, response to each scenario. Candidates are evaluated and scored on both the content and the manner of their preparation. The current criterion for passing, established by the certification committee, is 67%. An example of a common testing schedule and specific information about the three work-related stations of the practical examination is provided below.

Sample Practical Examination Schedule

The following rotation can occur in any order:

Business Planning Station (7 scenarios)	40 minutes	5-minute break
Staff Training (5 scenarios)	35 minutes	10-minute break
Situational Management (7 scenarios)	35 minutes	10-minute break

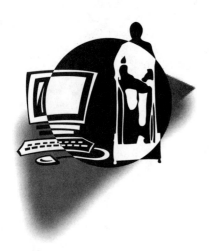

Business Planning Station

Candidates for the ACSM Health/Fitness Director® certification are expected to have a working knowledge and experience with respect to business planning. Regardless of whether the program is in a start-up period, maintenance mode, or expansion phase, business planning is essential for success. Each candidate for the ACSM Health/Fitness Director® certification will have the opportunity to respond to a hypothetical scenario requiring the use of business planning skills and knowledge. These business planning scenarios include, but are not limited to, such topics as budgeting, facility maintenance, operations, marketing, and program evaluation problems.

This section of the practical examination is composed of seven business planning scenarios drawn from one common business description. A general description of a health and fitness business is provided, and each business planning scenario will draw on this description to address a different aspect of the business planning process. The general business description is available to candidates 5 minutes prior to beginning the business planning scenarios. Candidates will have access to the general description during each scenario. Candidates have 2 minutes to read each scenario, craft a plan of action to solve the problem, and prepare to respond to the examiner. Candidates then have 3 minutes to present the scenario solution to the examiner. Examiners will then take 1 minute to score the response. This testing timeline will continue through each of the 7 scenarios.

Sample Business Description
You are the ACSM Health/Fitness Director® of a 100,000-square-foot, multipurpose commercial fitness center. The facility includes a pool, a gymnasium, cardiovascular and strength conditioning facilities, and racquetball courts. The facility is located in the suburbs of a large metropolitan area and has been in operation for 5 years. The club has four major departments: accounting and administration, membership services, health and fitness programs, and building services/maintenance. There is currently a staff of 65 employees (25 full-time, 32 part-time, and 8 contract). For the past 2 years, the membership has declined from 3,600 to 3,200 members, and the staff has been reduced to the present levels to accommodate the membership decline. The year-end financial statement reflects a break-even year, with total revenues of $2,750,000 (membership accounting for 85% of these revenues).

Sample Financial Planning Scenario
The general manager of the fitness center has just sent you a directive to find two areas in your operating budget in which expenses can be reduced with minimal impact on program delivery. Respond to this directive and defend your answers on the basis of data regarding the fitness center or the industry.

Note: Instructions to the Candidate: You are to read this scenario carefully for 2 minutes. You may ask the examiner to clarify the scenario; however, no interpretation or amplification of the scenario can be provided. You are to evaluate the conditions surrounding the management problem and respond to the request during a 3-minute period. You will be evaluated on both the manner and content of your response.

Situational Management Station

Candidates for the ACSM Health/Fitness Director® certification are expected to cope with unexpected problems in the day-to-day management of programs. Frequently, the solution to these problems requires directors to "think on their feet." This section of the practical examination is composed of seven situational management scenarios in which candidates have 2 minutes to read a scenario, craft a plan of action, and prepare to respond to the examiner. Candidates have 3 minutes to present the scenario solution to the examiner. The examiner will then take 1 minute to score the response. Candidates are scored on both the content of the response and the manner of presentation. This testing timeline will be repeated through all seven situational management scenarios.

Sample Situational Management Scenario

Your fitness manager has enrolled a member into the fitness program who should have been referred for further medical evaluation because of a risk factor related oversight on the member's health history questionnaire. The new member is the president of a local corporation who recently purchased 10 memberships for his senior managers. After a brief discussion with the member, he explains to you that he feels great and plans to continue following his 4-week-old fitness program with four visits a week in the center. How do you handle the situation?

Note: Instructions to the Candidate: You are to read this scenario carefully for 2 minutes. You may ask the examiner to clarify the scenario; however, no interpretation or amplification of the scenario can be provided. You should evaluate the conditions surrounding the management problem and respond to the request during a 3-minute period. You will be evaluated on both the manner and content of your response.

Staff Training Station

Candidates for the ACSM Health/Fitness Director® certification are expected to have a working knowledge of staff training and demonstrate the ability to effectively prepare staff on all aspects of program operations. The ACSM Health/Fitness Director® should

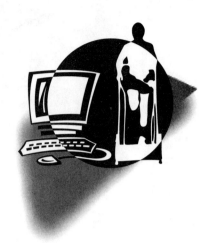

be able to develop job descriptions and training programs for a variety of positions within a fitness setting: front desk, fitness instructors, personal trainers, group exercise leaders, clerical and billing personnel, sales staff, pool staff, day care staff, housekeeping/maintenance staff, as well as supervisors and managers. The staff training component also addresses hiring, discipline and termination knowledge and skills. The candidate will be expected to review a variety of staff situations and provide responses that focus on high-quality customer service, safe and effective member care, and an understanding of policies and procedures based on a strong knowledge of the industry and profession.

This section of the practical exam is composed of 5 staff training scenarios involving various training opportunities. Candidates are given 3 minutes to review the scenario and develop a training outline to present to the examiner. Candidates then have 3 minutes to present their response to the examiner. The examiner will take 1 minute to score the response. Candidates are scored on both the content of the response and the manner of the presentation. This testing timeline is repeated through the 5 staff training scenarios.

Sample Staff Training Scenarios

You are conducting a staff training session with a new fitness instructor. You are to instruct them on their responsibilities regarding member service and member safety in the resistance training area. Outline the content of your training session addressing the importance of member service and safety, specific tasks that should be included in the training and methods of follow-up to ensure training was effective.

Instructions to the Candidate

You are to read this scenario carefully for 3 minutes and prepare your response. You may ask the examiner to clarify the scenario; however, no interpretation or amplification of the scenario can be provided. You should evaluate the conditions surrounding the management problem and respond to the request during a 3-minute period. You will be rated and evaluated on both the manner and content of your response.

■ **REFERENCES**

ACSM. *ACSM's Guidelines for Exercise Testing and Prescription.* 6th ed. Baltimore: Lippincott Williams & Wilkins, 2000.

ACSM. *ACSM's Resource Manual for Guidelines for Exercise Testing and Prescription.* 3rd ed. Baltimore: Williams & Wilkins, 1998.

ACSM. *Exercise Management for Persons with Chronic Diseases and Disabilities.*

Champaign, IL: Human Kinetics, 1997.

ACSM. *Health Fitness Facility Standards and Guidelines.* 2nd ed. Champaign, IL: Human Kinetics, 1997.

Chenoweth LS. *Worksite Health Promotion.* Champaign, IL: Human Kinetics, 1998.

Gerson RF. *The Fitness Director's Guide to Marketing Strategies and Tactics.* Champaign, IL: Human Kinetics, 1992.

Grantham WC, Patton RW, York TD, et al. *Health Fitness Management.* Champaign, IL: Human Kinetics, 1998.

Herbert D. *Legal Aspects of Preventive, Rehabilitative & Recreational Exercise Programs.* 3rd ed. Champaign, IL: Human Kinetics, 1997.

Heyward VH. *Advanced Fitness Assessment & Exercise Prescription.* 3rd ed. Champaign, IL: Human Kinetics, 1998.

Wilson BR, Glaros TE. *Managing Health Promotion Programs.* Champaign, IL: Human Kinetics, 1994.

Founded in 1954
AMERICAN COLLEGE of SPORTS MEDICINE®

Priscilla M. Clarkson, Ph.D.
President
University of Massachusetts
Amherst, Massachusetts

Angela D. Smith, M.D.
President-Elect
Children's Hospital of Philadelphia
Philadelphia, Pennsylvania

Barry A. Franklin, Ph.D.
Past President
William Beaumont Hospital
Royal Oak, Michigan

Barbara E. Ainsworth, Ph.D.
First Vice President
University of South Carolina
Columbia, South Carolina

Edward T. Howley, Ph.D.
First Vice President
University of Tennessee
Knoxville, Tennessee

W. Larry Kenney, Ph.D.
Second Vice President
Pennsylvania State University
University Park, Pennsylvania

Janet Walberg Rankin, Ph.D
Second Vice President
Virginia Tech
Blacksburg, Virginia

Russell R. Pate, Ph.D.
Treasurer
University of South Carolina
Columbia, South Carolina

James R. Whitehead
Executive Vice President
ACSM National Center
Indianapolis, Indiana

Street Address
401 W. Michigan St.
Indianapolis, IN
46202-3233 USA
Mailing Address
P.O. Box 1440
Indianapolis, IN
46206-1440 USA
Telephone
(317) 637-9200
FAX
(317) 634-7817
Web Site:
www.acsm.org
Federal I.D. Number:
23-6390952

**Advanced Team
Physician Course**
Nov. 30-Dec. 3, 2000
Orlando, Florida

ACSM Team PhysicianSM
Course Part II
Feb. 7-11, 2001
San Diego, California

**ACSM's Health & Fitness
Summit & Exposition**
April 17-20, 2001
Las Vegas, Nevada

ACSM 48th Annual Meeting
May 30-June 2, 2001
Baltimore, Maryland

MEMORANDUM

TO: *ACSM Health & Fitness Track Study Guide* Users

FROM: ACSM Committee on Certification and Education
Health/Fitness Track Subcommittee

SUBJECT: Updates to Study Guide

The following changes which have resulted from publication of the
ACSM's Guidelines for Exercise Testing and Prescription, sixth edition, should
be noted while preparing for the ACSM Group Exercise Leader$_{SM}$ and
ACSM Health/Fitness Instructor$_{SM}$ certification examinations.

Page 14
The Coronary Artery Disease Risk Factor table printed on page 14 of the
Study Guide has been updated in the 6th ed. of the *Guidelines*. Refer to page 24,
Table 2-1, in the 6th ed. of the *Guidelines* for the updated information to be used
on the certification examination.

Page 16, 51-52
The Initial Risk Stratification classifications printed on pages 16, 51-52 of the
Study Guide have been updated in the 6th ed. of the *Guidelines*. Refer to page 26,
Box 2-2, in the 6th ed. of the *Guidelines* for the updated information to be used
on the certification examination.

Page 52
The ACSM Recommendations for Medical Examination and Exercise Testing
Prior to Participation and Physician Supervision of Exercise Tests table printed on
page 52 of the *Study Guide* has been updated in the 6th ed. of the *Guidelines*.
Refer to page 27, Table 2-2, in the 6th ed. of the *Guidelines* for the updated
information to be used on the certification examination.

Page 40
In the Sample Questions/Answers printed on page 40 of the *Study Guide*, the
possible answers for question 19 should be: a. low risk; b. moderate risk;
c. high risk. The answer for question 19 is correct on page 41.

The committee appreciates your understanding of ACSM's ongoing quality
assurance and improvement process.